"Coaching has proven to be an essential tool fo
higher learning. Done right it will help solve pro
ieties face by students. Done well it can unleash h   , ... students.
This book is indeed timely as it provides some insights for those keen to
embark on the journey of coaching. I am confident existing and new practitioners of coaching will benefit immensely from this book. Congratulations
to the authors."

Professor Yaacob Bin Ibrahim, *Professor and Advisor to President,*
Singapore Institute of Technology, Former Ministers for Ministries of
Communications and Information (2011–2018), Environment and
Water Resources (2004–2011), Community Development
and Sports (2002–2004)

"This book clearly highlights the role of coaching, especially with a solutions focus, in readying students for their lifetime of learning. I like its
emphasis on the human touch, preparing the world of higher education for
what's most predictable about the future – it's unpredictability."

Paul Z Jackson, *co-author of* The Solutions Focus: Transforming
Change for Coaches, Leaders, and Consultants

"This book offers a holistic approach to coaching that will enhance student
learning, engagement and overall success. It is a comprehensive guide for
those interested in practical pathways which focuses on strengths, and foster
a positive and empowering approach to professional development. Plenty
of nuggets of wisdom for meaningful dialogues."

Simon TP Lee, *Accredited Master Executive Coach (AC),*
EMCC Global Accredited Master Practitioner (EIA),
Coach\Mentor Supervisor (ESIA)

"This is a book the world of HE sector has been waiting for: In depth,
insightful and innovative. The editors explore the key themes from group
work to PhD supervision, careers to internships to create an essential guide
for Higher Education coaching."

Professor Jonathan Passmore, *Henley Business*
School & EZRA Coaching

"Students in higher education today are faced with complex personal struggles, impacting their academic performance and growth. This invaluable book is a gem of resource for educators who wish to use coaching to enable and empower their students to tackle the various challenges they face. It provides varied scenarios and useful tips to guide faculty as they work with students individually and in groups. The systems perspective presented here is useful for educational institutions to consider as they plan to support student coaching and development holistically."

Josephine Teo, *EdD, MBA, PCC. ICF Singapore Board 2023–2024; Instructional Coach, Leadership Consultant and Coach, Certified Coach Supervisor*

"May Lim, Nadya Patel and Ramesh Shahdadpuri's excellent and timely contribution reminds us of the importance of the human connection in higher education. This is just what is needed right now. Highly recommended for anyone who supports students at university!"

Professor Christian van Nieuwerburgh, *Professor of Coaching and Positive Psychology, Centre for Positive Health Sciences, RCSI University of Medicine and Health Sciences.*

"This is a forward-looking and comprehensive book that highlights the importance of coaching in education in the 21st century. In this rapid changing world and the introduction of AI, the role of educators has evolved to be one that holds space for the development of students. I love how the emphasis is on the approach of using coaching to bring out the best to support the new generation for a better future."

Amily Ang, *President of International Coaching Federation (ICF) Singapore Chapter and Managing Director of The Growth Coach*

Coaching Students in Higher Education

This practical guide for educators in higher education encourages readers to ask effective coaching questions and apply relevant coaching techniques to empower and engage students to grow and perform at their best.

Filled with authentic examples and handy tips, the book takes readers from the "how to" of coaching, through the practicalities, challenges and honing of existing skills and new capabilities. The authors recognise that in educators' daily encounters and interactions with students, there are many timely coachable moments for authentic learning. These opportunities can enable students to learn beyond what is squarely in their curriculum and develop their own pathways to become work-ready graduates. Through coaching, educators help students discover more about themselves while guiding them to innovate and generate solutions to perceived and real-world problems. This guide offers in-depth discussions along with tools and tips to provide invaluable guidance for educators to get acquainted with the key skills needed to coach students for success in various academic and professional contexts. The content covers multiple varied scenarios, from classrooms and assignments, to internships and group work, and highlights various coaching opportunities with practical strategies.

This is a resourceful text for educators, teachers and professionals working in higher education and learning institutions. It provides training material for institutions that want to conduct faculty development programmes to prepare educators for effective coaching conversations in their universities.

May Sok Mui Lim an Associate Professor and Assistant Provost (Applied Learning) at the Singapore Institute of Technology (SIT). May is on a mission to promote coaching and transform the learning experience in higher education, and focuses on competency-based education, transition and improving learning. Recognised for her contributions, she received the National Day Honours: Public Administration Medal (Bronze) in 2022 and the SIT Teaching Excellence Award in 2016, 2019, and 2020. May is also an experienced occupational therapist by profession; she has been working with children with developmental delay and disorders in Singapore and Australia. A certified Solution-Focused Coach, she is dedicated to establishing a coaching culture for educators, aiming to develop students beyond the confines of the classroom.

Nadya Shaznay Patel is an Assistant Professor in the Business, Communication and Design cluster at Singapore Institute of Technology (SIT) and has over 20 years of experience as an educator, a researcher and trainer. With a passion for critical design futures thinking for interdisciplinary learning, she regularly facilitates workshops for educators and students. She recently published a journal article on Modelling Intellectual Empathy and Communicating Care. Committed to bridging the research–practice gap, she engages industry partners in applied research projects that leverage her expertise in Critical Design Futures (CDF)™ and interests in GenAI. Over the years, she has also worked with partners to offer industry-relevant workshops on empathetic leadership communication, personal branding and corporate coaching and mentoring.

Ramesh Shahdadpuri is an executive coach and educational development specialist with Singapore Institute of Technology (SIT). He leads coaching training and programmes for faculty development at the university for advancement of their professional capabilities as academics and in becoming effective educational leaders. Ramesh is a credentialed International Coaching Federation (ICF) coach and a Professional Certified Corporate Coach from Singapore Management University. He has served on the Board and Committees of ICF Singapore Chapter, and is an active member in various coaching communities of practice. His coaching practice and research interests include academic, leadership, positive psychology, solution-focused, supervision, team and youth coaching.

Coaching Students in Higher Education

A Solution-Focused Approach to Retention, Performance and Wellbeing

**Edited by May Sok Mui Lim,
Nadya Shaznay Patel and
Ramesh Shahdadpuri**

Routledge
Taylor & Francis Group

LONDON AND NEW YORK

Designed cover image: Getty

First published 2025
by Routledge
4 Park Square, Milton Park, Abingdon, Oxon OX14 4RN

and by Routledge
605 Third Avenue, New York, NY 10158

Routledge is an imprint of the Taylor & Francis Group, an informa business

British Library Cataloguing-in-Publication Data
A catalogue record for this book is available from the British Library

ISBN: 978-1-032-36470-4 (hbk)
ISBN: 978-1-032-36469-8 (pbk)
ISBN: 978-1-003-33217-6 (ebk)

DOI: 10.4324/9781003332176

Typeset in Times New Roman
by SPi Technologies India Pvt Ltd (Straive)

Contents

Foreword by Assoc. Prof. Nigel C. K. Tan

Coaching requires knowledge. It also requires experience, skill and importantly, requires an intrinsic desire to help someone else improve. It is not always easy to do it well. Yet, at a time when our students in higher education are grappling with change, it is vitally important that we as educators in the higher education domain do it consistently and do it well for the sake of our students. This is particularly important when dealing with heterogenous groups of learners in higher education – undergraduates, postgraduates, and adult learners – where coaching may require modification to suit the context and the learner.

I am thus delighted to see the publication of *Coaching Students in Higher Education: A Solution-Focused Approach to Retention, Performance and Wellbeing*. This book fills an important gap in the higher education context, not just for Singapore and Asia, but for educators all over the world. The three editors have assembled an A-team of experienced educators as authors, creating a book that successfully blends theory and practice. The book covers coaching in diverse higher education contexts – across different disciplines, across various environments – while emphasising the utility of coaching in these contexts. It offers clear solutions, providing useful frameworks undergirded by theory. It also remains very practical, using case vignettes to illustrate the authors' key points, and even providing sample questions and suggested responses to help those new to coaching. It does not shy away from confronting and acknowledging challenges to coaching, and it offers solutions for some challenging situations. In short, the focus on application is its greatest strength, and the book does live up to the title of being "solution-focused" indeed!

For the more experienced, it emphasizes the importance of recognizing coachable moments and reminds us all to pay attention not only to the cognitive but also the affective aspects of coaching. The book also takes an important step forward to consider coaching as a key strategy for a higher education organisation such as a university. Using a systems perspective, it asks us to consider what a coaching ecosystem might look like, how training for coaches might be operationalized and how to make it sustainable. It persuasively puts forth the case for coaching to be systematized, and it describes career paths for potential coaches. All these insights are relevant for educators anywhere in the world, which underscores the global applicability of these solutions.

Throughout these varied and diverse chapters, I was tremendously impressed not only by the logical organization of the sections but also by the quality of the content, and the consistency of the chapter formats and writing. Not only were the authors thoughtful and measured but the individual chapters were coherently linked through content, and through consistency, such as the use of case vignettes for all the chapters. This could only have come about through the efforts of the editors, who have gracefully walked the tightrope between theory and practice, and who have kept the practical aspects of coaching front and centre while maintaining the salience of theory.

I would thus like to congratulate both authors and editors for a splendid job in writing and editing this very valuable scholarly work. Like all good books, I hope this will prompt reflection in us as educators, and also inspire meaningful change in both individuals and organisations. At a time when higher education is buffeted by the winds of change and beset by a multitude of demands, this important book reminds us of our true purpose in education – that our goal is to help others improve, and that coaching remains a powerful tool for improvement for individuals and for organisations. I am confident that many in higher education, whether novice or expert, will find this book immensely helpful as a practical guide to coaching.

Assoc. Prof. Nigel C. K. Tan
Senior Consultant, Department of Neurology,
National Neuroscience Institute
Group Director Education (Undergraduate),
Singapore Health Services
Associate Dean, MD Programme,
Duke-NUS Medical School

Foreword by Dr Carol Kauffman

For the simplicity on this side of complexity, I wouldn't give you a fig. But for the simplicity on the other side of complexity, for that I would give you anything I have.

Oliver Wendell Holmes Sr

The future of education is here.

The ideal coach or coach trainer is one who is familiar with the theory, research, and practice. It is unusual to find authors who are well versed in all three. May, Nadya and Ramesh are uniquely skilled in their ability to translate coaching theory and research into the artful practice of a coaching mindset in education. They have combed the literature, drawn from diverse fields, best practices and woven them together seamlessly in a way that allows educators to implement the work in their day-to-day work with students. It is a paradigm shift in education.

The authors have indeed offered the readers "simplicity on the far side of complexity". The book is clear, illuminating, theoretically sound, pragmatic and quietly inspirational. They make the case for a coaching mindset in education but also guide the reader through the process, offer case examples, coaching dialogues and support all aspects of their work with sound theory and the latest research.

When reading the manuscript, I started taking notes to help me write the foreword. It didn't take long for me to start taking notes for myself. I can't say this book simply does an excellent job for educators to expand their teaching repertoire to include coaching. This is one of the best coach-training books I have ever read. As the Founder of the Institute of Coaching and an Assistant Professor at Harvard Medical School, I get sent many books, but it's been a few years since I've enjoyed one as much.

The world of work and of leadership has changed radically given the continuous escalation of disruption. Having a teacher capable of having coaching conversations empowers students on multiple levels. While it fosters psychological safety, creativity, performance and self-esteem, it also does more. Our next generation of leaders need to be equipped for the real world. Educators are powerful role models. As students experience teachers who can operate with a coaching mindset, they don't just learn that approach, they absorb it. It then becomes part of their internal operating system. By experiencing coaching at the outset of their careers these students start out with a crucial "soft skill" advantage. Most of the leaders I coach don't get held back by what they know or what they do. In a survey of 1,000 CEOs, with an annual revenue of 4 trillion dollars we asked, what feedback have you been told is your "Achilles Heel"? By far the challenge was their soft skills, listening, talking too much and not creating positive relationships. In other words, they lacked the crucial coaching mindset.

Having our future leaders "marinated" in a coach approach to learning can create a new wave of leaders equipped to face the never-ending changing world that requires agility, emotional intelligence and the capacity to create trusting relationships. What better way to do that, than to experience it?

There is a labyrinth of choices in any student – teacher interaction. What kind of relational-learning-emotional environment will the educator create? While it requires a shift in behaviours, it does not take "extra" time; in fact, it may save time. However, while inculcated habits are hard to break, the authors make it clear it is worth the time and effort. They take readers by the hand and walk them through the process and teach the skills and mindsets necessary to be successful.

In 2012, we began a Faculty as Coach program at Harvard Medical School. Every internal medicine resident was required to have a senior faculty as coach. A team of researchers followed the group over three years. They found that simply having three to four meetings a year with a faculty coach had a significant impact. We received Harvard Medical Schools Inaugural Award in Creating a Culture of Excellence. However, we had one result which may surprise you. Based on Richard Boyatzis' work on CEOs who coach their reports, we also asked the question, "Is coaching good for the coach?" During the tumultuous years of medicine, with demands of compliance with new regulations and mandated electronic records, physician burnout escalated. One group at Harvard Medical School did not experience burnout. These were faculty who were also coaches. As educators embrace this approach, not only will their students' careers and lives improve, but theirs will as well.

Carol Kauffman PhD
Founder, Institute of Coaching
Assistant Professor, Harvard Medical School
Thinkers 50, top 8 Global Coaches, 2019, 2023

Bibliography

Boyatzis, R. E., Smith, M. L., & Blaize, N. (2006). Developing sustainable leaders through coaching and compassion. *Academy of Management Learning & Education*, 5(1), 8–24.

Palamara, K., Kauffman, C., Stone, V. E., Bazari, H., & Donelan, K. (2015). Promoting success: A professional development coaching program for interns in medicine. *Journal of Graduate Medical Education*, 7(4), 630–637.

Palamara, K., Kauffman, C., Chang, Y., Barreto, E. A., Yu, L., Bazari, H., & Donelan, K. (2018). Professional development coaching for residents: Results of a 3-year positive psychology coaching intervention. *Journal of General Internal Medicine, 33,* 1842–1844.

Patton, D., & Herrera, G. (2021). "It Starts with the CEO: A Global Study, 2021," Egon Zehnder.

Contributors

Holly Andrews is an associate professor in Coaching and Behaviour Change at Henley Business School, United Kingdom, leading research and knowledge exchange for The Henley Centre for Coaching

Joe Chan is a youth life coach, founder and director at Ark of Hope Pte Ltd, Singapore

Eric Chern-Pin Chua is an associate professor and director of SIT Teaching and Learning Academy (STLA) at Singapore Institute of Technology, Singapore

Karina Dancza is an occupational therapist and associate professor at Singapore Institute of Technology, Singapore, who is passionate about lifelong learning and workforce development.

Bavani Divo is a senior educational developer at Singapore Institute of Technology, Singapore, who is dedicated to enhancing the educational experience through her work with students.

Fun Man Fung is an instructor at the National University of Singapore, Singapore

Rebecca J. Jones is a professor of coaching and behavioural change at Henley Business School, United Kingdom and co-founder of the Inclusive Leadership Company.

Boon Yong Kwok is a senior manager at Singapore Institute of Technology, Singapore, where he helps students to navigate the intricacies of the workplace.

Cheryl Pei Ling Lian is an academic adviser and assistant professor at the Singapore Institute of Technology, Singapore, where she empowers students to take ownership of their academic success through solution-focused coaching conversations.

May Sok Mui Lim is an associate professor and assistant provost (applied learning) at Singapore Institute of Technology, Singapore. She is also an occupational therapist and a solution-focused coach.

Valerie P. C. Lim is a speech therapist, and an associate professor and programme leader of the Speech and Language Therapy Programme at Singapore Institute of Technology, Singapore.

Kyrin Liong is an assistant professor of Engineering at Singapore Institute of Technology, Singapore.

Mara McAdams is a physician, coach and assistant professor at Duke-NUS Medical School, Singapore.

Chee Ming Ong is a lead educational developer at Singapore Institute of Technology, Singapore.

Gin Yong Ong is a career coach at Singapore Institute of Technology, Singapore.

Nadya Shaznay Patel is an assistant professor of design innovation at Singapore Institute of Technology, Singapore, where she endeavours to make thinking skills explicit for students through intellectually empathetic and dialogic coaching conversations.

Ramesh Shahdadpuri is an executive coach and educational development specialist at Singapore Institute of Technology, Singapore.

Rendell Kheng Wah Tan is a senior lecturer at Singapore Institute of Technology, Singapore.

Jeffrey Guan Ching Thng is a career educator at Singapore Institute of Technology, Singapore where he helps students to develop essential career skills and prepares them for a smooth transition from university to the workplace.

Peng Cheng Wang is an associate professor in the Engineering Cluster and deputy director of SIT Teaching and Learning Academy (STLA) at Singapore Institute of Technology (SIT), Singapore.

Weili Zhang is a career educator at Singapore Institute of Technology, Singapore, where she helps students to build their personal brand and be career ready.

Preface

What an enriching and edifying experience it has been working on this book. We came together with a clear goal: to illustrate why coaching is essential in higher education. Throughout our careers, we have seen that education should be more than just an academic pursuit and achievement. It is about developing the whole person – intellectually, emotionally and socially. We recognise that education should not just be about transmitting disciplinary content knowledge but nurturing the whole person. This belief is the cornerstone of our work and the essence of this book.

In academia, we often witness a focus predominantly on intellectual growth. However, we understand that true development extends far beyond this. It encompasses the nurturing of emotional, mental, and spiritual health. Attributes like empathy, analytical skills and critical thinking are not just supplementary; they are essential to forming a well-rounded individual. This understanding aligns with how scholars define whole-person development, which emphasises the holistic growth of a person's actions and behaviours rather than solely their knowledge acquisition.Our shared passion for coaching stems from our belief in its power to transform students' educational experiences. The book explores how coaching can help students grow in all aspects of life. Our approach is informed by a simple yet profound understanding: students are more than their grades. They are individuals with unique challenges and aspirations. Our goal is to empower educators to use coaching to help students become autonomous, resilient, and ethical members of society.

Embarking on a solution-focused approach to coaching dialogues, our collaborative intent is for readers to skilfully navigate and elevate their effectiveness in supporting students' holistic development. By incorporating a myriad of higher education contexts where coachable moments naturally unfold, our vision is for educators to embrace opportunities that enable students to flourish. We aspire to instil in educators the joy and privilege inherent in guiding students through their distinctive challenges and aspirations, reinforcing the essence of whole-person development that underpins our collective journey in this book.

In crafting this book, we aim for it to be both a practical guide and a source of inspiration for everyone – educators, coaches and supervisors alike. We express our heartfelt thanks to the chapter authors whose shared dedication exemplifies the strength of common goals. By sharing our stories and insights, we hope to spark a passion for nurturing students' overall growth through coaching. Special thanks to our colleague Tam Yew Chung for his unwavering support in keeping us on course. Our commitment is to transform higher education into a space that fosters all-around development, not just for careers but for life. We invite readers to join us in this pursuit.

Tell me and I forget
Teach me and I remember
Involve me and I learn
Coach me and I discover
    Inspired by Confucius

Part I

The What, Why and How of Coaching in Higher Education

1 Coaching in Higher Education

Creating Impact

May Sok Mui Lim and Nadya Shaznay Patel

Chapter Objectives

- To identify the key factors driving the increasing relevance of coaching in higher education, including the changing landscape and the growing importance of transferable skills.
- To examine the role of coaching learning theories and how they can be applied in higher education.
- To discuss the importance of creating a coaching ecosystem within higher education institutions and fostering a culture encouraging coaching conversations among educators and students.
- To emphasise the potential long-term impact of coaching on student success, wellbeing, and educator–student relationships in higher education settings.

Keywords

coaching culture
coaching ecosystem
coaching mindset
educator–student relationship
student relationship
student success
student wellbeing
trust
wellbeing

> Tell me and I forget, teach me and I remember, involve me and I learn, coach me and I discover.
>
> Inspired by Confucius

DOI: 10.4324/9781003332176-2

Introduction

This chapter sets the stage for understanding the relevance and impact of coaching in higher education. It begins by defining coaching and differentiating it from other developmental practices, such as mentoring, advising and counselling. It provides an overview of existing coaching practices in higher education, highlighting their increasing significance as educators strive to develop students holistically, beyond mere content knowledge delivery. The chapter then highlights the role of coaching and learning theories and the importance of building trust and rapport in coaching relationships. It also emphasises the need for a coaching mindset, key coaching skills, and competencies. Next, we discuss the importance of creating a coaching ecosystem within higher education institutions, encouraging a culture where coaching conversations are widely understood and practised. We urge educators and institutional leaders to commit to building a supportive coaching culture that benefits academics, students and staff alike. We sought to highlight educators' pivotal role in students' lives and demonstrate how coaching can enhance the educator–student relationship, ultimately improving student success and wellbeing. By examining the current research, practices and future directions, this chapter provides a complete perspective on the potential of coaching to create a lasting impact in higher education.

Evolving Landscape of Higher Education

Current Global Trends

The higher education landscape is transforming significantly as the world adapts to the rapid digitalisation and automation of Industry 4.0 and the knock-on effects of the COVID-19 pandemic. The traditional model of providing students with knowledge and skills through an undergraduate programme to prepare them for a lifelong career is no longer sufficient to meet the demands of today's job market. The World Economic Forum (WEF) highlighted four key challenges facing higher education in 2019 (Østergaard & Nordlund, 2019), including the need for lifelong learning, changing student expectations, the impact of digital disruption on learning and education business models, and the shift towards valuing skills over degrees. Since then, the pandemic has further accelerated these changes, and we are now seeing a significant shift in how we live, work and learn. These socioeconomic changes significantly impact the education sector, and educational institutions must adapt to meet these new demands.

As the demands of the modern workforce continue to evolve, higher education institutions face increasing pressure to adapt their teaching methods and curricula to better prepare students for the future. The World Economic Forum's 2022 report on Catalysing Education 4.0 highlights the need for inclusive and lifelong education opportunities, with learners taking greater responsibility for their skill-building and career development. To meet these changing expectations, educators must shift away from a traditional, teacher-centric approach and instead act as facilitators and enablers of student learning. This requires rethinking the traditional education model, including moving from lecture-based instruction to focusing on hands-on, experiential learning and experimentation with emerging technology like Generative Artificial Intelligence (GenAI) tools. Aoun (2017) proposes that a 'robot-proof' education system does not feed students facts but reconditions their minds and develops new skills for creativity and inventiveness, qualities of high societal value. Additionally, universities must consider alternative forms of assessment and measurement, such as competency-based assessments, to reflect better the knowledge and skills needed to succeed in today's rapidly changing workforce.

Impact on Education

Learners have more learning choices and can pick up knowledge from alternative education providers, mainly through digital and hybrid platforms. With the availability of high-quality bite-size learning materials, the rise of corporate universities, and the proliferation of industry certificates and innovative online learning tools, there is an urgency to rework the higher education model and promote more effective and impactful ways of educating learners, especially for knowledge and skills in high-growth industries and promising emerging sectors.

Transdisciplinary learning is gaining prominence in higher education due to its capacity to provide students with a comprehensive and multifaceted grasp of intricate issues that cannot be thoroughly explored through a single disciplinary lens. As the future becomes more complicated and intertwined, graduates need the skills to navigate multiple domains and viewpoints and collaborate efficiently with individuals from various backgrounds (Ehlers, 2020). Transdisciplinary learning fosters this ability and provides students with valuable transferable skills, such as critical thinking, problem-solving, and communication, that are highly valued in the workforce (Ehlers & Eigbrecht, 2020). Transferable skills refer to relevant skills and abilities across different professions, enabling individuals to move from one job to another. They are essential for professional work and are also relevant socially and for lifelong learning.

As the economy becomes more volatile and jobs are disrupted or transformed with the rise of automation and artificial intelligence, the role of universities in developing students' transferable skills alongside technical skills becomes more important. While technical skills can be acquired through knowledge acquisition and training, transferable skills are better cultivated through experience and coaching. In higher education, educator–student coaching provides a dynamic, interactive environment that encourages students to reflect on their learning, engage in active problem-solving and develop effective communication strategies. Through coaching, educators can guide students in identifying their strengths and areas for improvement, setting realistic goals, and fostering resilience and adaptability in the face of challenges.

By actively participating in coaching conversations, students acquire transferable skills and learn to apply them in diverse contexts, enhancing their overall preparedness for the evolving professional landscape. Finally, while tools may be developed for AI-enabled coaching, this book focuses on the human touch for coaching students, where interactions are focused on social and emotional connections with a physical presence for verbal and non-verbal communication skills.

Understanding the Concept of Coaching

What is the essence of coaching? Sir John Whitmore rightly and concisely said, "Coaching unlocks people's potential to maximise their performance" (2017, p. 12). What better place to unlock people's potential than the university?

Coaching, as defined by Cox et al. (2014), is "a human development process that involves structured, focused interaction and the use of appropriate strategies, tools and techniques to promote desirable and sustainable change for the benefit of the coachee and potentially for all stakeholders" (p. 1). Despite varying definitions of coaching, coaching is most commonly viewed as an approach to individual learning and development, characterised by the unique features that differentiate it from other learning and development interventions.

It is worth highlighting the fundamental difference between a directive or telling and a non-directive or asking type of communication. The former is where the communicator provides specific instructions, guidance, or information to the receiver, rarely or without seeking input. On the other hand, the latter is a style where the communicator asks open-ended questions, actively listens and encourages the receiver to participate in the conversation. See Table 1.1.

Overall, the choice between directive or telling communication and non-directive or asking communication depends on the specific goals of the conversation, the needs of the student, and the context of the situation. A skilled educator can use both communication styles effectively to support their students' learning and development. A coaching conversation that involves asking questions and encouraging discovery rather than direct telling would be more effective in maximising a student's potential.

Table 1.1 Difference Between Directive or Telling and Non-Directive or Asking

	Directive or telling	*Non-directive or asking*
Communicator's role	Provides specific instructions or information	Asks open-ended questions and actively listens
Receiver's role	Receives information or instructions	Participates in the conversation and provides input

Coaching is more than just asking good questions. A good coaching conversation through reflective inquiry involves reflective statements and questions to trigger people to reflect on their thoughts (Reynolds, 2020). In the book *Coach the Person, not the Problem*, Reynolds (2020) highlights the importance of developing the person rather than solving an immediate problem. Beyond asking questions, coaching involves noticing energy shifts, playing back the individual's beliefs and assumptions, summarising complex outcomes and possibilities, offering observation when an individual shows resistance and reflecting on the progress of growth. Good coaching is not always comfortable. This is because learning often happens in moments of uncertainty, especially when we begin to doubt the beliefs and assumptions we have been making and explore different perspectives (Reynolds, 2020).

Many educators or leaders may think that it is easier or quicker to give advice, share a solution or provide an answer rather than taking the time and effort to coach someone to get to the solution. While offering advice or solutions may be quick and efficient, it risks making people depend on those with more experience for answers or approval before they act (Reynolds, 2020). In the long run, people may lose the motivation to think for themselves, and providing advice will not result in independent thinkers. Individuals who are not after advice may hear or forget or not act on the solution provided. When we tell people what to do, their short-term memory is activated, and that is where learning is least effective. On the other hand, coaching requires tapping into people's prior knowledge to consider a new way forward, arousing more motivation, creativity and a positive sense of responsibility. It facilitates insight-based learning, creating new awareness and perception change (Reynolds, 2020).

The other approach worth highlighting is mentoring and counselling. Mentors are often more experienced and established individuals with similar backgrounds or expertise to their mentees. Often, mentoring focuses on providing guidance, advice, and support to students based on the mentor's experience and knowledge. While coaching focuses on the present and future, mentoring focuses on the past and present, sharing insights and wisdom based on personal experience (Inzer & Crawford, 2005). While both coaching and mentoring can be valuable forms of support in higher education, coaching is typically more focused on skill development and performance improvement. At the same time, mentoring often relates to career development and professional growth (Giacumo et al., 2020).

On the other hand, counselling is a therapeutic process aimed at addressing emotional, psychological or behavioural issues affecting a student's wellbeing or academic performance (Bachkirova & Baker, 2018). Counsellors help students gain insight into their feelings, thoughts and behaviours, and they may develop coping strategies or offer recommendations for treatment if necessary. When an educator or coach identifies a student with mental health and personal wellbeing issues, one should refer the student to a professional counselling service. Although there may be some overlap in the goals and methods of coaching, mentoring and counselling, it is essential to recognise their distinct roles and tailor the support provided to meet the needs of individual students best.

While this book focuses on coaching, an effective educator can navigate between the roles of a coach, a mentor or an instructor. Counselling should be provided by a professionally trained counsellor depending on what a student needs and the goals and outcomes the student hopes to achieve; a skilled educator can decide which approach to take. We avoid an overly prescriptive approach to determining when to coach, mentor or instruct.

Coaching within the Context of General Education

Coaching in education has grown and attained greater visibility over the last two decades in schools and higher education institutions, especially in Australia, Europe and the United States. The term "coaching in education" embraces a range of interventions and practices in educational settings, involving students, educators and other stakeholders to improve outcomes for learners and transform learning ecosystems.

Campbell and van Nieuwerburgh (2018, p. 5) developed a global framework for coaching in education. The framework takes a holistic view of the educational coaching ecosystem and consists of four key contexts:

•   Educational leadership
•   Professional practice
•   Community engagement
•   Student success and wellbeing

Details of the four contexts are shown in Table 1.2.

The global framework takes a holistic view of the educational coaching ecosystem, recognising that coaching can support the development of leaders, professionals, and communities, as well as the success and wellbeing of students. The model is designed to be open, inclusive and adaptable, and can serve the needs of diverse types of learning institutions. Each pillar can be seen as a portal or entry point. An institution thinking of implementing coaching can start with any of these elements as a point of entry and gradually expand to the others in creating a sustainable coaching ecosystem. The focus of our book will be on coaching students for their success and wellbeing.

One aspect of coaching in education is *instructional coaching*, pioneered by Jim Knight from the University of Kansas. Knight (2007) considers instructional coaching an approach with the primary objective of refining teaching practices and boosting student learning outcomes. The emphasis is placed on professional development and support for educators, in which the coach assumes the roles of a partner, advisor and mentor. Knight asserts that successful professional development entails one-on-one interactions, active listening, empathy, open dialogue and candid communication (2007). This aligns with the "Professional practice" pillar of Campbell and van Nieuwerburgh's (2018)

Table 1.2 The Global Framework for Coaching in Education

Educational contexts	Description
Educational leadership	Coaching supports the development of educational leaders who can inspire and motivate their teams, build relationships and create a culture of continuous improvement. Coaching can help leaders develop skills in areas such as communication, collaboration and decision-making.
Professional practice	Coaching supports the ongoing development of teachers and other education professionals, helping them to reflect on their practice, identify areas for improvement and develop strategies for growth. Coaching can help professionals develop skills in areas such as classroom management, pedagogy and assessment.
Community engagement	Coaching supports the development of strong relationships between schools and the wider community, helping schools to engage parents, community organisations and other stakeholders in the educational process. Coaching can help educators develop skills in areas such as communication, relationship-building and community outreach.
Student success and wellbeing	Coaching supports the development of strategies to promote student success and wellbeing, helping educators to identify and address the needs of individual students. Coaching can help educators develop skills in areas such as differentiated instruction, social-emotional learning, and student engagement.

global framework. Specifically, it refers to coaching educators to be successful in teaching so that the student achieves success (Hasbrouck & Michel, 2021). In instructional coaching, the goal is to provide effective and strategic professional development and learning to teachers to improve student outcomes. Unlike instructional coaching, which focuses on developing teacher's classroom practices and pedagogy, this book will focus on coaching students or learners, specifically in higher education.

Growing Relevance of Coaching in Higher Education

In the context of higher education, coaching is emerging as an increasingly significant and impactful approach for fostering effective learner development. Educators should re-evaluate their perceptions of teaching and explore the inclusion of coaching in their pedagogical "toolbox". The following are some key reasons why incorporating coaching is essential.

Types of Learners

First, the types of learners coming to university are more diverse, with varied demographic profiles and personal backgrounds. The traditional 18 to 21-year-old high school leavers can benefit from coaching to reflect and discover strategies or solutions that can work in the university environment. The mature learner brings a wealth of work and life experience and can be coached to draw upon them when dealing with academic tasks and challenges. The first-in-the-family learners may not have someone in the family to learn from in terms of transitioning, coping or learning effectively in a university. Understanding the needs of the different groups of learners, an influential educator can coach them to find the best solutions and way forward towards their goals.

Coachable Moments

Second, a "teachable moment" refers to an unplanned opportunity to provide a specific lesson or insight, and a "coachable moment" is a planned or unplanned opportunity for a coaching conversation focused on supporting an individual's growth and development in a specific area, such as decision-making or problem-solving. Many spontaneous coachable moments exist within and outside of the curriculum hours. When students struggle in decision-making or problem-solving a challenge, instead of immediately offering advice, an educator can reach out and offer a coaching conversation to support them. More can be found in Chapter 3. Beyond the academic context, coachable moments may also occur within an internship at the workplace and are discussed in Chapter 9. Employers increasingly recognise the value of interpersonal skills, adaptability and emotional self-awareness in navigating today's complex professional landscape. Coaching can help students develop these crucial abilities, better preparing them for the challenges they will face in their careers. An educator can work closely with workplace supervisors to coach students, integrating what is learnt in the university to workplace challenges.

Educator–Learner Relationship

Third, the coaching relationship is built on trust and respect. Educators, whether as professors, teaching assistants, academic coaches or career coaches, can help students they look up to for learning and guidance. When students seek help, they can use coaching to empower the learners to discover solutions, take action, and remain accountable. With coaching, it enables the educator to get to know the learner better and continue to build relationships and trust. Moreover, coaching plays a pivotal role in fostering inclusive learning environments. By adopting an empathetic coaching approach, educators can create safe spaces for students from diverse backgrounds to express their thoughts, opinions and experiences. This is discussed in depth in Chapter 4.

High Tech, High Touch

Fourth, with the proliferation of online learning tools and artificial intelligence in higher education, students increasingly spend time in the virtual learning environment. Students need to feel more connected to the learning community. The more "high tech" that higher education becomes, the more "high touch" educators need to be to engage with learners. As teaching can become more efficient with online materials or learning packages, educators can spend more time providing feedback and coaching students to meet their learning goals. Educators can also use different online tools and dashboards to help identify at-risk students who may benefit from more coaching, as discussed in Chapter 6.

Current Coaching Practices in Higher Education

Coaching is increasingly relevant in higher education because it provides a personalised, strengths-based approach to support students in achieving their goals and overcoming challenges. It is focused on developing self-awareness, improving performance and enhancing overall wellbeing. By providing individualised support, coaching can help students reach their full potential so they will succeed academically and professionally.

In higher education, several coaching approaches address various needs, including one-on-one coaching and group coaching models. One-on-one coaching models involve personalised coaching sessions between a coach and a student, tailored to the student's specific needs, goals, and challenges. This individualised approach fosters a deeper understanding of the student's capabilities, strengths, and growth areas, promoting targeted skill development and problem-solving strategies. Group coaching models, on the other hand, bring together students with similar goals or interests, facilitating peer learning and collaboration while still offering the guidance of a coach. This approach provides a supportive environment for students to share their experiences, ideas and challenges, fostering collective growth and development. This is discussed in depth in Chapter 7.

For managers and emerging leaders seeking to prepare themselves for career advancement further, coaching is often embedded in business school Master of Business Administration (MBA) curriculums to support the development of their leadership, communication, problem-solving and strategic thinking, and differentiate themselves in the workplace (Hall & Towell, 2016; Steiner et al., 2017). Coaching can be embedded in various forms, such as providing students access to executive coaches, incorporating coaching skills training into coursework, or offering coaching sessions as part of an experiential learning component. Furthermore, some MBA programs may include a coaching practicum or internship, where students can practise their newly acquired coaching skills by working with real clients.

Another area where we see coaching occurring is in career coaching. Career coaching involves supporting students and recent graduates in their career development and helping them prepare for the workforce. Beyond the coaching conversations to help students develop a clear vision of their ideal career path, career coaches may also guide job search strategies, networking, resume and cover letter writing, interview preparation, and identifying career paths that align with the student's skills, interests and values. By working with a career coach, students can better understand their strengths, weaknesses, and goals, and identify specific actions they can take to achieve their desired outcomes for work. Chapter 11 of this book goes in-depth on career coaching.

Another application of coaching is the use of successful coaches in the typical curriculum of a competency-based education (CBE) programme. Success coaches primarily assist with student-specific needs by creating individual development plans and milestones to address academic and non-academic concerns (Chow et al., 2023; Robinson & Gahagan, 2010). An extensive literature on CBE has found that learners greatly benefit from success coach support regarding academic and social integration and a sense of belonging (Brower et al., 2017; Rainwater, 2016). These benefits likely result from the validation, affirmation and individualised attention provided to the learner by the success coach (Robinson, 2015). In addition to coaching conversations, success coaches may support students in effectively navigating appropriate resources and practising new skills, resulting in performance improvement and increased persistence in studies.

More can be done to incorporate coaching in universities' undergraduate and other degree programmes. Coaching students goes beyond imparting knowledge in a traditional classroom setting. It is an effective method for developing skills and abilities. By viewing coaching as an extension of hands-on learning, educators can have regular, meaningful conversations with their students and focus on fostering engagement, enlightenment, and empowerment to support their holistic development and readiness for the workforce (Hesseln & Gair, 2016).

The Intersection of Coaching and Learning Theories

Coaching is a highly effective approach to learning that helps individuals reach their personal and professional objectives. Griffiths (2015) draws on education research and her Coaching Learning Model, comparing the coaching process and learning stages. According to Griffiths (2015), coaching in the context of learning involves working collaboratively with a coach and typically begins with establishing learning goals. It is followed by tasks described as the three learning stages: Discovery, Application and Integration (Griffiths & Campbell, 2009), as illustrated in Table 1.3.

In the learning context, the natural outcome of coaching is gaining self-knowledge. This highlights the role of cognitive strategies in coaching. When coaching becomes a continuous and iterative process, self-knowledge becomes woven into the learning process, enabling the learners to rise beyond their immediate learning goals and create a self-directed learning environment. Metacognitive strategies also play a significant role in coaching, as they involve the process of learners reflecting on their thinking, learning, and problem-solving approaches. Through coaching, students can develop metacognitive skills such as self-assessment, self-regulation and planning.

Table 1.3 Learning Coaching Model

Learning stages	Coaching process involves
Discovering New knowledge	• Listening • Relating • Questioning • Reflecting
Applying New knowledge	• Accountability • Action
Integrating New knowledge	• Self-coaching • Taking responsibility

Source: Griffiths and Campbell (2009).

These skills allow learners to monitor their progress, evaluate their learning strategies, and adjust their approaches accordingly, fostering a greater sense of ownership and autonomy.

Coaching fits in well with adult learning theories. One which is proposed by Mezirow (1990, 2000, 2018), transformative learning theory, describes learners as having learning experiences that can produce shifts in thinking and significantly impact learners' future experiences. It mainly focuses on adult education and young adult learning, which fits well with the students we work with at the university. Adults construct frames of reference from their experiences throughout life that guide their behaviour and mindsets. These frames of reference typically inhibit one from considering other perspectives that deviate from or contradict our rigid preconceptions. When adults face challenges against their frames of reference, it results in them questioning their effectiveness and opportunities are created for coaching conversations, which can lead to transformation (Cox, 2015). Therefore, informed by transformative learning theory, coaching can aim at supporting learners to gain awareness of ineffective frames of reference and move towards perspective transformation. Coaches provide a safe and welcoming environment for preconceptions to be challenged and an opportunity to explore and assess alternative perspectives (Cox, 2015).

The above discussion underscores the importance of tailoring coaching approaches to learners' unique needs and contexts, recognising their prior experiences, motivations, and goals. It also highlights the potential for coaching to facilitate profound, transformative learning experiences, ultimately contributing to the holistic development of learners and creating an impact in higher education.

Research Studies on Coaching in Higher Education

In addition to the theories, increasing research studies look into coaching in higher education (Devine et al., 2013; Fried & Irwin, 2016; Hesseln & Gair, 2016). For example, Lancer and Eatough (2018) designed a qualitative study to investigate the effects of coaching on undergraduates. Students were interviewed at different time points to share their coaching experience. The authors found that coaching provided a platform for undergraduates to address a range of common issues, such as time and stress management, confidence and interpersonal skills. Coaching gave students increased control over their studies and other areas, improved their ability to balance and focus, increased their confidence levels and helped them see new perspectives on various issues.

Coaching was also found to help support learners transitioning between professional and academic life. Spencer (2021) studied non-traditional students' coaching experiences during their undergraduate education using a heuristic inquiry approach. Three themes emerged from students' accounts. First, students felt coaching offered a non-judgemental and comfortable space for open dialogue. Although apprehension and scepticism may surface initially, coaching conversations can be used to connect with students and establish a working relationship to encourage open discussions during coaching sessions. Second, students reported increased motivation, awareness of emotions, and decreased stress levels after coaching. Last, Spencer (2021) lamented that a consistent struggle reflected implicitly or explicitly during coaching sessions with many non-traditional students was the issue of confidence; many portrayed low levels of confidence in their academic ability and themselves. However, despite these overall positive accounts of students' coaching experiences, the sample of non-traditional students included various profiles of learners, and how these learners' experiences with coaching differed due to their specific needs still unresolved.

In the field of education, there is a growing body of research that supports the use of coaching as an effective tool for enhancing learning and development. Despite the various coaching philosophies and methods available, successfully integrating a coaching approach requires active participation from key stakeholders, including students, educators and leaders. By fostering a collaborative and supportive environment, these parties can drive transformative change and establish a new learning culture in which individuals and organisations adopt a coaching mindset and approach to teaching and learning. (Devine et al., 2013).

Critical Components for Successful Coaching: Mindset and Relationship Building

Beyond the theories and research studies that support coaching in higher education, we believe the most essential ingredients for successful coaching boil down to mindset and relationships. Coaching can help students to believe in themselves and know that their success is due to their efforts. This means that students must also know that educators believe in them and that they are empowered, supported, and encouraged to make their own decisions. The mindset that educators bring is vital.

Consider these three statements: (i) *I think this person is a problem*; (ii) *I think this person has a problem*; (iii) *I think this person is on a learning journey and has the potential to grow*. Each of these statements evolves a different response to the conversation that we may have with the person. Bringing a coaching mindset means that, as educators, we refrain from being judgemental but rather see potential in our students, especially when they are making mistakes or having problems.

Positive relationships and rapport between educators and students are essential for positive coaching outcomes in higher education. This is because students are more likely to engage in the coaching process and be open to feedback and guidance when they feel supported, trusted and respected by their educators.

However, shifting from an instructor to a coach mode can be challenging for many educators in higher education. Educators are often trained to be experts in their fields and to be directive and authoritarian in their teaching approach. In contrast, coaching requires a more collaborative approach, requiring the educator to adopt a curious mindset to guide on the side, supporting the student's discovery rather than the expert in the room.

To successfully adopt a coaching approach, educators must be willing to adapt and develop new skills, such as active listening, open-ended questioning and non-judgemental feedback. This requires a shift in mindset from one of authority to one of partnership, where the educator works alongside the student as a co-learner and co-creator.

With enough like-minded educators who believe in adopting a coaching approach, a community can be formed to support each other in improving coaching skills and discovering best practices. A coaching ecosystem in higher education can then be built to establish a new learning culture in which individuals and organisations adopt a coaching mindset and approach to teaching and learning.

Conclusion

This chapter began by providing an overview of the changing landscape in higher education. We defined coaching and compared it with direct instruction and mentoring. Before its relevance and application in higher education, we discussed coaching in the general education context. We then explored coaching and learning theories before discussing research studies on coaching in higher education. With this introduction, we hope readers have gained a good overall perspective of what exists in the literature, education landscape and higher education. Importantly, before concluding, we highlighted that shifting from an instructing mode to a coaching mode can be challenging, but it is essential for promoting positive outcomes in higher education. Changing mindsets and building relationships are essential ingredients for effective coaching in higher education to enable students to achieve their goals and reach their full potential.

References

Aoun, J. E. (2017). *Robot-proof: Higher education in the age of artificial intelligence*. The MIT Press. https://doi.org/10.7551/mitpress/11456.001.0001

Bachkirova, T., & Baker, S. (2018). Revisiting the issue of boundaries between coaching and counselling. In S. Palmer, & A. Whybrow (Eds), *Handbook of coaching psychology* (pp. 487–499). Routledge. https://doi.org/10.4324/9781315820217-40

Brower, A. M., Humphreys, D., Karoff, R., & Kallio, S. (2017). Designing quality into direct-assessment competency-based education. *The Journal of Competency-Based Education, 2*(2), e01043. https://doi.org/10.1002/cbe2.1043

Campbell, J., & van Nieuwerburgh, C. (2018). *The leader's guide to coaching in schools: Creating conditions for effective learning*. Corwin. https://doi.org/10.4135/97815063 35841

Chow, P. C., Matius, J., & Lim, S. M. (2023, 13 September). *How to coach in-employment lifelong learners for success*. Times Higher Education. www.timeshighereducation. com/campus/how-coach-inemployment-lifelong-learners-success

Cox, E. (2015). Coaching and adult learning: Theory and practice. In J. P. Pappas, & J. Jerman (Eds), *Transforming adults through coaching: New directions for adult and continuing education, number 148* (pp. 27–38). Wiley Periodicals. https://doi.org/10. 1002/ace.20149

Cox, E., Bachkirova, T., & Clutterbuck, D. (Eds). (2014). *The complete handbook of coaching*. SAGE Publications.

Devine, M., Meyers, R., & Houssemand, C. (2013). How can coaching make a positive impact within educational settings? *Procedia: Social and Behavioral Sciences, 93*, 1382–1389. https://doi.org/10.1016/j.sbspro.2013.10.048

Ehlers, U.-D. (2020). *Future skills: The future of learning and higher education*. Springer. https://doi.org/10.1007/978-3-658-29297-3

Ehlers, U.-D., & Eigbrecht, L. (2020). Reframing working, rethinking learning: The future skills turn. *Proceedings of the European Distance and E-Learning Network (EDEN) Conference, 1*, 1–10. https://doi.org/10.38069/edenconf-2020-ac0001

Fried, R. R., & Irwin, J. D. (2016). Calmly coping: A motivational interviewing via co-active life coaching (MI-VIA-CALC) pilot intervention for university students with perceived levels of high stress. *International Journal of Evidenced Based Coaching and Mentoring, 14*(1), 16–33.

Giacumo, L. A., Chen, J., & Seguinot-Cruz, A. (2020). Evidence on the use of mentoring programs and practices to support workplace learning: A systematic multiple-studies review. *Performance Improvement Quarterly, 33*(3), 259–303. https://doi.org/ 10.1002/piq.21324

Griffiths, K. (2015). Personal coaching: Reflection on a model for effective learning. *Journal of Learning Design, 8*(3), 14–28. https://doi.org/10.5204/jld.v8i3.251

Griffiths, K., & Campbell, M. (2009). Discovering, applying and integrating: The process of learning in coaching. *International Journal of Evidence Based Coaching and Mentoring, 7*(2), 16–30.

Hall, D., & Towell, M. (2016). Exploring the value of executive coaching to MBA students at the University of Portsmouth Business School. *HR Bulletin: Research and Practice, 10*, 7–9. https://researchportal.port.ac.uk/en/publications/exploring-the-value-of-executive-coaching-to-mba-students-at-the-

Hasbrouck, J., & Michel, D. (2021). *Student-focused coaching: The instructional coach's guide to supporting student success through teacher collaboration*. Paul H. Brooks Publishing Co.

Hesseln, H., & Gair, J. (2016). Bridging the gap between higher education and the workforce: A coach approach to teaching. *Philosophy of Coaching: An International Journal, 1*(1), 63–79. https://doi.org/10.22316/poc/01.1.06

Inzer, L. D., & Crawford, C. B. (2005). A review of formal and informal mentoring: Processes, problems and design. *Journal of Leadership Education, 4*(1), 31–50. https://doi.org/10.12806/v4/i1/tf2

Knight, J. (2007). *Instructional coaching: A partnership approach to improving instruction.* Corwin Press.

Lancer, N., & Eatough, V. (2018). One-to-one coaching as a catalyst for personal development: An interpretative phenomenological analysis of coaching undergraduates at a UK university. *International Coaching Psychology Review, 13*(1), 72–88. https://doi.org/10.53841/bpsicpr.2018.13.1.72

Mezirow, J. (1990). *Fostering critical reflection in adulthood: A guide to transformative and emancipatory learning.* Jossey-Bass.

Mezirow, J. (2000). Learning to think like an adult. In *Learning as transformation: Critical perspectives on a theory in progress* (pp. 3–33). Jossey-Bass.

Mezirow, J. (2018). Transformative learning theory. In K. Illeris (Ed.), *Contemporary theories of learning* (2nd ed., pp. 114–128). Routledge. https://doi.org/10.4324/9781315147277-8

Østergaard, S. F., & Nordlund, A. G. (2019). *The 4 biggest challenges to our higher education model – And what to do about them.* World Economic Forum. www.weforum.org/agenda/2019/12/fourth-industrial-revolution-higher-education-challenges/

Rainwater, T. S. M. (2016). Teaching and learning in competency-based education courses and programs: Faculty and student perspectives. *The Journal of Competency-Based Education, 1*(1), 42–47. https://doi.org/10.1002/cbe2.1008

Reynolds, M. (2020). *Coach the person, not the problem: A guide to using reflective inquiry.* Berrett-Koehler Publishers.

Robinson, C., & Gahagan, J. (2010). Coaching students to academic success and engagement on campus. *About Campus: Enriching the Student Learning Experience, 15*(4), 26–29. https://doi.org/10.1002/abc.20032

Robinson, C. E. (2015). *Academic/success coaching: A description of an emerging field in higher education* [Doctoral thesis, University of South Carolina]. Scholar Commons. https://scholarcommons.sc.edu/etd/3148/

Spencer, D. (2021). Understanding the coaching experiences of non-traditional students in Higher Education in the UK. *International Journal of Evidence Based Coaching and Mentoring, 15*, 84–95. https://doi.org/10.24384/00V3-NM61

Steiner, S., Dixon, D. P., & Watson, M. A. (2017). MBA coaching program: Best practices for success with limited resources. *Management Teaching Review, 3*(1), 86–97. https://doi.org/10.1177/2379298117723315

Whitmore, J. (2017). *Coaching for performance: The principles and practice of coaching and leadership* (5th ed.). Nicholas Brealey Publishing.

World Economic Forum. (2022). *Catalysing education 4.0: Investing in the future of learning for a human-centric recovery.* www.weforum.org/reports/catalysing-education-4-0-investing-in-the-future-of-learning-for-a-human-centric-recovery/

2 Coaching for a Preferred Future

The Solution-Focused Approach

*May Sok Mui Lim, Joe Chan and
Ramesh Shahdadpuri*

Chapter Objectives

- To identify key principles and ideas of the solution-focused coaching approach.
- To discuss the benefits of coaching students towards their preferred future, moving away from thoughts and behaviours linked to their troubled past or dreaded future.
- To examine practical solution-focused techniques.
- To discuss common concerns educators have when using solution-focused coaching and how to overcome them.
- To highlight the issue of ethics and boundaries for educators, including knowing when and how to refer students for further professional help beyond the scope of coaching.

Keywords

goal orientation
GROW
preferred future
resource activation
resourceful past
scaling
SCORE
solution talk
strengths

> The best way to predict the future is to create it.
>
> Abraham Lincoln

DOI: 10.4324/9781003332176-3

Introduction

This chapter will explore key principles, ideas and practices of the solution-focused approach in coaching. We share the advantages of taking a forward-looking perspective, especially with young adults like students in higher education, as they make important decisions related to their academic and personal development, career choices, and life after graduation.

Origins of the Solution-Focused Approach

The solution-focused approach originated in the field of family therapy in the 1980s. It was developed by Steve de Shazer, Insoo Kim Berg and their colleagues at the Brief Family Therapy Center in Milwaukee, Wisconsin. Unlike traditional therapeutic interventions that view a person's challenges as problems and deficiencies, with the need to determine causation and take remedial steps to overcome them, the solution-focused approach is based on the belief that people have innate resources and abilities to solve them (de Shazer et al., 2007). The role of care providers is to help clients identify, build and leverage their resources and strengths to move forward rather than focusing on past problems.

De Shazer and Berg were influenced mainly by the giants in psychotherapy, like Milton Erickson (1901–1980), who emphasised the importance of focusing on the present and future rather than the past. Another significant influence was Gregory Bateson (1904–1980), whose work in anthropology and linguistics stressed the importance of focusing on solutions rather than problems. De Shazer and Berg found that positive language was crucial in the desire to change. When clients engaged in solution talk and spoke about hope and possibilities, they were energised. When trapped in problem talk and negativity, clients become depressed and would fall into a gloom-ridden cycle (Green & Palmer, 2018).

De Shazer and Berg developed an *Interactional View* in their solution-focused approach, with a focus on the here and now rather than depending on the client assessments done in the past (Jackson & McKergow, 2007). They intended to help shift the client's mindset towards a better future by building on what already worked well and identifying resources and strengths mediated by positive language. Solution-focused has emerged as a strengths-based approach that draws on an individual's resources and resilience to seek pathways for making positive change. This approach has become accepted in various helping professions, including therapy and coaching (Grant et al., 2012).

Key Principles and Themes of the Solution-Focused Approach

Solution-focused coaching is a strengths-based, outcome-oriented method that emphasises what is working rather than what is not. The approach is based on the belief that individuals can be empowered to make positive change with accessible resources and innate abilities to solve problems by focusing on solutions rather than diving into the root causes of the problem. We begin with a coaching vignette and introduce student Jay and Professor M in Box 2.1.

The solution-focused approach has a positive disposition that can help someone discover what is working. We can use solution-focused approach to have coaching conversations with students. Solution-focused practice draws on a fundamental set of principles, which are listed below as summarised by Campbell and van Nieuwerburgh (2018):

- Finding the root cause does not always help
- Focus on the preferred future
- If something works, do more of it
- If something does not work, try something else
- People can be very resourceful

Box 2.1   Introducing Jay

Jay: Hi, Prof M! It's Jay here. I got my results today and am thankful for your coaching session last semester. Will you be free next week for a quick follow-up session?

Four months have passed since Jay had a coaching conversation. Jay is a first-year health science undergraduate student. She took a gap year after high school to work before starting university. When Jay first met Prof M, she was burdened and disappointed after receiving her grades from her first semester. She needed to figure out how to better cope with the academic work and the multiple demands of part-time work.

Jay has always done well in balancing her academic and commitments outside school. She wondered what had gone wrong in university and whether she had made the wrong choice of course to study.

Prof M is a busy professor with a heavy teaching load and numerous research projects. Jay asked to speak to her to discuss what to do with her disappointing results. Prof M knew that setting aside time for the conversation with Jay was important. Moreover, it had to be a time-effective, impactful conversation that could help her student.

Prof M used a solution-focused approach, which helped to shift the student's mindset from a negative to a hopeful one. Jay made good progress in the next semester and asked for a follow-up coaching session.

Finding the Root Cause Does Not Always Help

Identifying the root cause of a problem is optional to help someone find a solution. Some believe it is important to analyse the problem thoroughly before solving it. However, we should appreciate that there are varying degrees of complexity in every problem. Furthermore, a situation may be confidential, and the individual may not be comfortable sharing too much. Situations involving people rarely unfold logically and predictably, and some cases may need to be urgently addressed. Therefore, the solution-focused approach can minimise the time and effort spent investigating the problem while seeking to understand the context and focusing on exploring the preferred future.

Focus on the Preferred Future

This involves spending more time looking forward rather than thinking about the past. When we focus on problems and shortcomings, switching from problem talk to solution talk takes greater effort, which can help generate possibilities and spur optimism. Focusing on the preferred future instead of what has gone wrong generates vibrancy and positive energy. Solution talk creates accountability and encourages one to explore constructive ideas, while problem talk can lead to a blame game and a greater sense of hopelessness (Lee, 2021). Some people dwell on their troubled past, mistakes and the negativity they experienced. However, conversations of the troubled past fosters rumination and generate more negative energy, veering away from a sense of hope and new possibilities. While it can be hard to imagine and consider their preferred future, shifting the person's focus to an ideally different future would help create positive energy and potential solutions.

If Something Is Working, Do More of It

It is important to appreciate that everyone's problem is different and unique. What works for someone may be different for another. Helping the person discover what has worked in the past or even what is working now amidst challenges can provide clues that lead to potential solutions. There could be things that are already working but seem inadequate or camouflaged by other things going wrong. Therefore, a conversation to unpack what is already working or has worked in the past raises morale and hope, and reminds the individual of their capabilities.

If Something Does Not Work, Try Something Different

Humans are creatures of habit. We can trap ourselves by repeating mistakes which reoccur in different guises. There is great value in helping a person discover what needs to change. Sometimes, what seems to be working are "stop-gap" measures which bring temporary relief to a bigger chronic problem. For example, taking a nap in the middle of the day may help a sleep-deprived student to function and get by, but it is unsustainable if he regularly stays up to 3 a.m. to complete his work. Discovering what is not working, deciding to stop and making a change with something different can help create new insights and yield positive outcomes.

People Can Be Very Resourceful

Coaching conversations can start with "problems" a person brings up. The key to a fruitful solution-focused conversation is identifying the individual as a resourceful and capable person who can make changes for themselves. This differentiates coaching from the pathological therapy approach in recognising that individuals are resourceful and able to seek and own solutions to their problems. We only need to help them uncover it.

Understanding the Characteristics and Needs of Young Adults

Before we go further into solution-focused coaching, it is essential to understand the profile of our learners. While the profile of learners in higher education is getting more diverse, many learners are young adults. We know that today's youth have grown up in a rapidly changing world, developing unique characteristics shaped by their environment and experiences. Understanding who they are and their needs will help educators to engage them effectively and have coaching conversations to support their goals. Here are some positive characteristics that are commonly associated with this group of young adults:

- Tech-savvy digital natives
- Global-minded and politically aware
- Diverse
- Independent
- Resilient

Tech-Savvy Digital Natives

They are tech-savvy as they have grown up with technology and use it pervasively in their daily lives. They are exposed to new technology trends and adopt them quickly. The speed of information and ease of access is much faster than the generations before; when it comes to problem-solving, they usually turn to the internet for answers or crowdsource solutions from friends through social media. They may also turn to generative artificial intelligence to seek solutions. When coaching them, the real need is for the coach to guide them to discover solutions that specifically address them as individuals rather than providing generic solutions such as good time management habits.

Global-Minded and Politically Aware

Today's youth have access to global information and worldwide perspectives. This has helped create a more globally minded generation and awareness of the world's interconnectedness. Their worldviews are no longer limited to what authority figures in their lives tell them. At the same time, many appreciate the value of coaching and mentoring and receiving sincere, valuable feedback.

Diverse

Today's youth are more aware of diversity than ever before. Knowledge of various ethnicities, religions, cultures and other backgrounds represented in society has led to a greater understanding and acceptance of different perspectives and ways of life. It is usual for today's youth to navigate spaces with ambiguities, in-betweens and relativism rather than absolutes. When coaching and solution-finding, educators must be comfortable that solutions young adults identify with may differ greatly from what they would have chosen.

Independent

Young adults today are growing up and living in a world with unprecedented access to information and resources than ever before. They are a generation who are more independent, self-reliant and able to make their own decisions. However, when they feel overwhelmed, vulnerable and lost, they may seek help and guidance, asking for more directions before picking themselves up and being independent again. Therefore, how they prefer to receive information and communicate is a personal choice that each one decides independently. As a coach, empowering them to seek more information, make decisions, take action and be accountable will help to build their confidence and independence.

Resilient

Today's youth have grown up in a world where the pace of change is much faster than previous generations. They are capable and well-equipped to adapt to new circumstances and external challenges. However, they could experience dissonance, and we can observe if their inner states have genuinely caught up with all the external changes. Providing opportunities to explore in safe spaces to try out ideas and even fail will help them learn and grow. As coaches, even if we foresee that their solutions may not work, we can support and help them build resilience.

Why Solution-Focused Approach Works Well in the Higher Education Context

Coaching can be used in education settings to complement traditional teaching methods to help students achieve academic goals and develop life skills, such as time management and emotional regulation. Coaching can help educators improve their instructional practices and develop leadership skills in themselves and the students. When we interview educators who care for their students, their number one concern about using coaching to support their students' success is time. Other concerns include not wanting to spoon-feed their students with solutions, and fear of uncovering and dealing with issues educators do not feel equipped to handle. These worries can be addressed if educators understand more about coaching and the benefits of the solution-focused approach.

Educators are often challenged with the multiple demands of academia, the common ones being teaching, marking, conducting research, writing publications, grant applications and administrative work. Hence, time becomes a very precious commodity. Solution-focused coaching can be time-effective for educators by not spending too much time on the past and focusing instead on present realities and future possibilities. Educators should avoid conversations discussing the troubled past, such as why the student was not confident as a child, what created the "fear for Maths" or specific personality issues contributing to negative team dynamics. It usually takes too long to unpack them, and more significantly, we are not in a position to fix the past. Dwelling on the troubled past is unhelpful as it cannot be undone. Solution-focused coaching conversations can help students reflect and leverage their resourceful past, make the most of their present and find pathways to reach their preferred future. While it is essential to understand the situational context, the focus should be on spending time and effort to support the student's goals and solutions for success.

On the concern of spoon-feeding students, solution-focused coaching advocates the opposite approach. Instead of giving them instant advice or solutions, students are seen as resourceful individuals who can be coached and empowered to discover what solutions work for them and the actions they want to take. With proper communication of expectations, educators can set the ground rules and boundaries of the coaching relationship, focusing on coaching for academic progress and personal development, not personal relationships, financial issues or mental health struggles. Setting clear expectations helps the students understand what they will receive coaching on. Educators can be equipped with information and resources to direct students who need support beyond their ambit, such as counselling and financial assistance. When necessary, the educator can guide the learners in solution-focused coaching towards proactively seeking appropriate support, such as making an appointment with the counsellor.

Solution-Focused Perspectives from the Academic and Practitioner Lens

We have shared about the characteristics of young adults today and why solution-focused coaching works well in higher education. This section looks at the "how" of the solution-focused approach. Insights from researchers and practitioners and examples of various coaching techniques and solution-focused questions will be discussed. Readers new to coaching are encouraged to develop further insights into solutions-focused coaching by attending coaching training and practising the coaching techniques. After all, developing coaching competency takes practice and feedback.

Solution-Focused Coaching Conversations

Moon describes coaching as "a dialogic process that constructs the notion of purpose, possibility and progress" (2020, p. 247). The coach–coachee conversation is a collaborative process that helps the coachee in meaning-making. When appropriate words and language are used, the coach plays a big role in helping the coachee achieve greater awareness and be motivated to change for the better. The Dialogical Orientation Quadrant (DOQ) is a conversational map that the coach can use to guide the coaching conversations and steer them towards the coachee's preferred future, away from fear of the troubled past or the dreaded future (Moon, 2020).

Solution-focused coaching is highly pragmatic with minimal application of concepts. The coach uses solution-seeking language and techniques in conversations with the coachee (Green & Palmer, 2018). After the coachee becomes aware of his realities, assumptions and best hopes, the coach guides the coachee to identify available resources, discover strengths and explore preferred outcomes. The coachee then determines the actionable steps to move forward and succeed.

Coaching for Performance Outcomes

A motivated individual can work with a coach to support him in his quest to progress from where he currently is to achieve a higher level of performance. In solution-focused coaching, Grant (2011) identified three key contributing factors for a coachee's performance improvement and progress towards their preferred desired outcome:

- Goal orientation – the coachee determines his preferred outcomes, works on developing viable solutions, and commits to positive action.
- Resource activation – the coach helps the coachee to identify and use strengths and to activate personal, social and organisational resources to move forward with purpose.
- Problem disengagement – the coach supports the coachee to shift away from past problems and setbacks and to focus on the present and future instead, directing efforts to their preferred outcome and goal attainment process.

A coach has the flexibility and free choice in using various solution-focused tools and techniques. The coach–coachee conversations will always come around to goal orientation, resource activation and problem disengagement, which are the central tenants of the solution-focused coaching approach.

Solution-Focused Coaching Techniques

The following are helpful techniques for solution-focused coaching drawn from a practical handbook by Lee (2021):

- Coach the person, not the problem – Even if the coachee is ranting about their problems, the coach must focus beyond the actions and behaviours. Draw the coachee to their inner self and innate resources to raise their self-awareness and develop capabilities.
- Allowing space to think – Reflecting and developing awareness takes time. The coach must be comfortable with silence and allow the coachee to respond without being rushed.
- Use the coachee's language – Using language familiar to the coachee makes the coachee feel listened to and respected. This is especially important for educators who may tend to use education and industry jargon. For example, regarding managing distractions, a question like "Why do you think self-regulation is important?" can be too difficult for a student to understand. Using more straightforward language and familiar words is more helpful for clarity and understanding.
- Listen, select, build – This is a very effective technique of listening and turn-taking for creating a quality conversation that drives towards the coachee's preferred future – by listening for what is truly important for the person, then selecting and building on it. Enables the conversation to move toward what the coachee cares about.

Solution-Focused Coaching Questions

In a coaching conversation, the coach may ask various questions to get the coachee to think and explore. The SCORE questions serve as a good guide on the different types of questions a coach can consider asking (Lee, 2021). SCORE is an acronym for Scaling, Confidence, Outcome, Relationship and Exception. Here is a walkthrough of when and how to use these coaching questions.

- Scaling – Scaling questions are helpful for coachees to develop perspectives of where they currently are and where they wish to move towards. Scaling can help the coachee to visualise and get clarity of the subject. It is easy to use and is very versatile. Scaling questions can help surface hidden assumptions, what is already working, and to imagine what improvement looks like. Examples of scaling questions include:
  - On the scale of 1 to 10, with 10 representing your ideal outcome and 1 being the opposite, where are you now?
  - What is already working for you to be at this point on the scale?
  - Suppose you moved one point higher; what difference would you notice?

- Confidence – Confidence questions, as the name suggests, aim to build confidence and self-belief by illuminating capabilities and positive aspects of the situation to the coachee. They help the coachee identify the aspects that are working, raise hope and encourage them to take a step forward. Some examples of confidence questions include:
  - How have you managed to get this far?
  - What personal strengths and successful past experiences can help you achieve the desired outcomes?
  - What could give you more confidence and positive support to take action towards your preferred future?

- Outcome – Outcome questions are good for clarifying the goal and desired state the coachee is striving for. They are used for drawing out behaviour-based outcome goals. They are important, especially when a coachee may rant and complain but needs clarification on what they want and hope to achieve. Some examples include:
  - Suppose the issue we are discussing today is resolved; how would things be different?
  - Which of the different things you have in mind is the most important to address in working towards your preferred future?
  - What would be some positive effects of reaching your desired outcome?

- Relationship – Relationship questions encourage the coachee to consider solutions from an outsider's perspective. These questions can be beneficial, especially if the coachee seems to have a narrow or limited view of the context or possible solutions. It invites the coachee to explore more widely, consider others' perspectives, and gain new insights. Examples of relationship questions include:
  - Consider a person with a different perspective on this issue; what would this person say?
  - Suppose someone knows you well and wants you to succeed; what would this person suggest?
  - Who else may have some similar experiences that you can learn from?

- Exception – Exception questions help to develop awareness that no problem happens all the time. Even when things are very difficult, there may be potential solutions within the problem. Exception questions are beneficial for coachees who are very negative or feel hopeless about a situation. Such questions encourage them to reframe, identify contrary situations and generate new ideas to move forward. Some exception questions include:
  - Looking back to when things were better, what did you do then that you may consider trying again now?
  - Please share the most recent example of when you were at your best, even in a small way.
  - What might you notice if the situation has improved, even by a little bit?

In addition to these exception questions, the coach can also consider asking the "miracle question". It takes a bit of imagination but can be very helpful in gaining insights on how the coachee would like to see themselves if they were free of their problems. An example goes like this:

- Suppose … that you wake up tomorrow, a miracle has happened. All the problems you raised were resolved. You did not know that the miracle occurred since you were sound asleep. As you go about your day, what would you discover? How would you know the miracle happened? What would you observe? How would you react differently?

Asking the miracle question is a pleasant invitation to visualise and imagine. It takes curiosity and skills from the coach to follow up with questions and help the coachee to shift and discover plausible actions that bring reality closer to the imagined future.

Using GROW Model to Frame a Solution-Focused Conversation

Learning to ask a variety of coaching questions is helpful but insufficient. Coaching involves skills to conduct an intentionally managed conversation, and it is important to frame the coaching conversation so that the dialogue between coach and coachee flows effectively. The GROW model (Whitmore, 2017) is a widely adopted in coaching and from our experience in introducing it to educators in our university, the framework is easily understood and appreciated to guide and a facilitate a coaching conversation. GROW is an acronym for Goal, Reality, Options and Way Forward as shown in Figure 2.1.

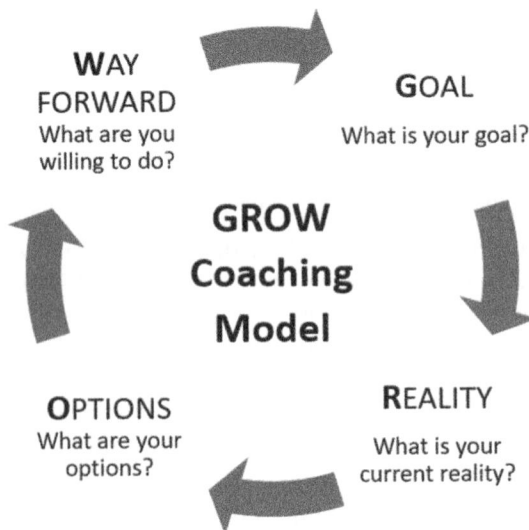

WAY FORWARD
What are you willing to do?

GOAL
What is your goal?

GROW Coaching Model

OPTIONS
What are your options?

REALITY
What is your current reality?

Figure 2.1 GROW model steps

Step 1: What Is Your Goal?

Imagine hopping into a taxi and asking to driver to drive, without telling the destination. It will lead nowhere or to a place you do not wish to be at. Similarly, a coach should always work to get the coachee to identify goal that they want to work towards. It is quite common that individuals know what they want to get away from or to overcome the problem that is bothering them, but they may not have a clear actionable goal. Therefore, it is important to spend some time in the coaching conversation trying to understand what the coachee hopes to achieve and articulate their desired outcome.

Some useful questions that we can ask at this stage are:

- What are you hoping to work towards?
- What would you like to achieve from today's conversation?
- What is your preferred future for the situation that you are talking about today?

Step 2: What Is the Reality?

While we want to avoid going into the troubled past to look for the root causes of a problem, it is essential to understand the context and assess the situation. Understand the current situation in terms of the actions taken so far. Clarify the results of actions previously taken, what has worked and what has not. It is also helpful to understand any obstacles and available resources. Resources can be previous successful experience, individual strengths, and people or assets that are accessible. Here are examples of questions you can ask:

- Share with me what has been happening ... what went well?
- Tell with me more about what you have tried so far.
- What similar situation did you encounter in the past and managed overcome it?
- How did your family, friends, and support group play a part in helping to get to where you are today?

Step 3: What Are Your Options?

Work with the individual to identify the possibilities and options. Keep going beyond the first one or two, no matter how good the options may sound. Explore strategies for making that option work. Help the coachee imagine and consider that the option is being trialled; what would they notice if it is working? Some questions you can ask are:

- I noticed that you could do that on your own ... how did you manage it?
- What are you learning from what you have just shared in our conversation?
- What would someone who knows and cares for you suggest you do?

- Suppose you were to increase your score by just one point on the scale, what needs to happen?
- Suppose you tried that option; what would you start noticing if it worked?

Step 4: Way Forward – What Will You Do?

As the session ends, the coach gets the coachee to summarise and share their understanding and learnings at this step. The coachee can summarise action plans for implementing the identified steps. It helps to create accountability by defining actions, timeframe and measures of progress. The coachee may also identify an accountability partner or other ways of showing commitment to the agreed action. Examples of coaching questions are:

- What actions and small steps will you choose to start with?
- How do you plan to follow through on what you have set out to do?
- If there is one thing you can start doing differently, what would it be?
- How confident are you in completing these actions to achieve your goal?

In Box 2.2, we continue with the vignette of a coaching conversation we introduced at the earlier part of the chapter.

In this vignette, the coach uses the GROW framework to navigate the conversation. We can observe that the student started negatively, describing herself as a failure, but progressively became more positive with the solution-focused coaching. Instead of dwelling on the negativity, the coach skilfully led the student to explore the reality of what was working before exploring options that the student could consider moving forward.

Box 2.2   Coaching Conversation between Jay and Prof M Using the GROW Model

Prof: What brings you here today, Jay?
Jay: Hi Prof, I have received my grades from the first semester. They were terrible. I am disappointed and am wondering what to do about it.
Prof: I see. I can sense your disappointment. The first year in university can be challenging.
Jay: You can tell me what I need to do differently to do better.
Prof: I am sure you are a resourceful student. I can't quite tell you what to do, but let us see if I can help you discover for yourself some way forward.
Jay: Yes, any way forward not to do so badly will be helpful.

Prof:	What would you like to take away from our conversation today for it to be helpful?
Jay:	Some strategies to study better or manage my time well may be helpful. **(Goal)**
Prof:	Help me understand how you spent your time in the first semester. **(Reality)**
Jay:	You see, I have always been good with my studies in high school. I juggled my time well with different activities such as dance, working part-time and still did well in my studies. However, it seems different now.
Prof:	It is good that you have done well in the past. Tell me more.
Jay:	Well, that was the past. I see myself as a failure now. Not only am I doing poorly in my studies, but I am also making mistakes in the different jobs that I am doing. It is like a different me altogether.
Prof:	Tell me about your different jobs. What are they?
Jay:	Well, my whole Saturday is spent running enrichment classes for young children. On Tuesday and Thursday evenings, I work at Starbucks. On Sunday, I continue to give tuition to a secondary school student I have worked with for the past two years. I realise I am making more mistakes, such as keying the wrong order and calling the children by the wrong names.
Prof:	Are you comfortable sharing the reasons for working three different jobs?
Jay:	My family doesn't need the money. I just enjoy doing different things. I like to be financially independent, too. Well, I worked a whole year like this before I entered university. I have already cut my Starbucks schedule from five to two evenings. Oh, for my enrichment class job, I hope that it can bring more experience to the course I am studying now.
Prof:	How have you been finding time to study? **(Reality)**
Jay:	Well, it is mainly the three weekday evenings. I am so exhausted on Sunday afternoon that I don't want to do anything else but rest.
Prof:	From what you understand from the curriculum, how many self-learning hours are recommended outside the timetabled hours?
Jay:	Interesting, I never really calculated them.
Prof:	Hmm, how about sharing what you have tried so far that works? **(Reality / Options)**
Jay:	When I reduced the Starbucks hours, I found that I created some time to revise and meet up with groupmates for the group work. But it may be insufficient. You got me curious; I should

determine how many hours I need for self-study in each module. And multiply it by the four modules that I am taking.

Prof:　Good thinking! What else? **(Options)**

Jay:　For one of the subjects I did well, I created a study plan on the topics to revise each week. Surprisingly, though that was the most challenging module, I didn't do too badly.

Prof:　Interesting … what does that insight suggest? **(Reality)**

Jay:　Hmmm … maybe if I set aside time and plan for revision, I can do better

Prof:　How do you propose to make time for all the modules? **(Options)**

Jay:　Honestly, I don't need to work so many jobs. Maybe I can pick them up again during the school holidays. Perhaps I can let go of the Starbucks evenings. Alternatively, I'll cut down my hours supporting the enrichment class. I need to work out my hours more carefully.

Prof:　Let us explore what else you can do to create more time for revision. **(Options)**

　　[The conversation continues …]

Jay:　Well, I am beginning to feel that I am not useless after all. I may have overcommitted and underestimated the time I need to set aside.

Prof:　What steps will you take to follow through on our discussion? **(Way Forward)**

Jay:　First, go back to my module profiles and calculate the required self-study hours in each module. Then, I should work out the hours I have left to do a job or two that I enjoy. I need to reassure myself that I can always do the jobs again during the school holidays.

Prof:　How will you make sure that you follow through? **(Way Forward)**

Jay:　Ha ha, I have a best friend; I should share with her and ensure she checks that I have done this. Oh, I also need to create a study plan, not just for the challenging module but for all of them.

Prof:　It sounds like you have a few actionable steps to work on.

Applying the Solution-Focused Approach in Everyday Educational Settings

In our experience working with students in educational institutions, we have encountered several challenges that educators commonly face. To arrive at a favourable outcome, we share our thoughts and practical handles on interacting with them differently.

Common Challenge Number 1: Doing Badly in Studies Yet Active in Extracurricular Activities

Sometimes, we see students who are very involved and enthusiastic in outside activities but are not interested in class. Sometimes, they even win trophies and medals, yet fail in their subjects. For such students, having a solution-focused coaching conversation could start with a curious stance where we learn to uncover their motivations and passion for these activities. Help them reconnect with the reasons and purpose for why they decided to enrol for their studies. As we uncover their positive attributes in those settings, we can affirm them for those characteristics and strengths they possess. By taking the time and effort to listen and understand them, we may discover that all it takes is to have an adult show interest in their lives and offer guidance on balancing their commitments.

Common Challenge Number 2: Easily Distracted and Lack Perseverance When Faced with Setbacks

Often, when things are moving very quickly for students to manage deadlines, assignments and projects, it is not uncommon for some of them to get side-tracked from their work. With a solution-focused coaching approach, we can help them manage their time and break down big goals and outcomes into smaller steps; we can help them be accountable by keeping track of time and activities together. It makes it more achievable when we ask what is needed for them to improve by just another point on their scale.

Common Challenge Number 3: They Appear Rude and Disrespectful Towards the Authorities and Rules

The solution-focused practitioner believes that individuals have potential and something that is already working well. It is the educator's job to highlight and amplify that. Hence, working with students this way puts them at ease and willing to be open to working on areas they need to improve. Helping young adults discover perspectives of how others view their actions and behaviours can shed light on how others may respond differently. Recalling how this generation of young adults embrace different values and appreciate diversity and inclusivity, helping them to realise and respect diverse values that differ from theirs can be favourable for their growth and development.

In regular interactions with students, we can share constructive feedback and highlight areas they are doing well in, strengthening our collaborative relationship with them.

Conclusion

In our interaction with students in higher education settings, we can use and advocate the solution-focused coaching approach to help them thrive in their university life and for the world of work when they graduate. While we know that a student's journey will not be a bed of roses, we can achieve much more by developing them holistically and building strong foundations. We can support them to discover and leverage their strengths, broaden their perspectives, and spark creativity in seeking innovative solutions. Whether our role is that of an educator, coach, mentor, advisor or administrator providing care and support, using a solution-focused approach, a "language of hope", can make a positive difference in our interactions with students to help them discover new possibilities and pathways.

Discussion Starters

- When you reflect on your current mindset and conversational style, how similar or different do you think it is from the solution-focused principles and characteristics highlighted in this chapter?
- What are some ways to learn and practice solution-focused conversational skills? How do you see yourself using them for effective dialogue with students, professional peers, work colleagues and your social circle?
- If a student you are coaching spends a lot of time talking of the past and ruminating, how can you reframe and shift the conversation towards having a more constructive coaching session?
- When is it a good opportunity in a coaching conversation to use scaling questions to help your student gain awareness and explore their preferred future? Think of some examples of good scaling questions you could use.

References

Campbell, J., & van Nieuwerburgh, C. (2018). *The leader's guide to coaching in schools: Creating conditions for effective learning.* Corwin. https://doi.org/10.4135/978150 6335841

de Shazer, S., Dolan, Y., Korman, H., McCollum, E., Trepper, T., & Berg, I. K. (2007). *More than miracles: The state of the art of solution-focused brief therapy.* Haworth Press.

Grant, A. M. (2011). The solution-focused inventory: A tripartite taxonomy for teaching, measuring and conceptualising solution-focused approaches to coaching. *The Coaching Psychologist, 7*(2), 98–106. https://doi.org/10.53841/bpstcp.2011.7.2.98

Grant, A. M., Cavanagh, M. J., Kleitman, S., Spence, G., Lakota, M., & Yu, N. (2012). Development and validation of the solution-focused inventory. *The Journal of Positive Psychology, 7*(4), 334–348. https://doi.org/10.1080/17439760.2012.697184

Green, S., & Palmer, S. (2018). Positive psychology coaching: Science into practice. In S. Green, & S. Palmer (Eds), *Positive psychology coaching in practice* (pp. 1–15). Routledge. https://doi.org/10.4324/9781315716169-1

Jackson, P. Z., & McKergow, M. (2007). *The solutions focus: Making coaching and change simple* (2nd ed.). Nicholas Brealey Publishing.

Lee, S. T. (2021). *Solution focused briefly illustrated*. Partridge Publishing Singapore.
Moon, H. (2020). Coaching: Using ordinary words in extraordinary ways. In S. McNamee, M. M. Gergen, C. Camargo-Borges, & E. F. Rasera (Eds), *The Sage handbook of social constructionist practice* (pp. 246–257). SAGE Publications. https:// doi.org/10.4135/9781529714326.n24
Whitmore, J. (2017). *Coaching for performance: The principles and practice of coaching and leadership* (5th ed.). Nicholas Brealey Publishing.

3   Identifying Coachable Moments

May Sok Mui Lim and Ramesh Shahdadpuri

Chapter Objectives

- To highlight essential coaching skills for educators to apply.
- To identify different encounters that educators can have with students in higher education settings for coaching conversations within and outside timetabled teaching hours.
- To explain the concept of "coachable moments" and "decision opportunities".
- To explore the decision on whether to inform students that they are being coached.
- To share examples of "coachable moments" and "decision opportunities" with case scenarios to illustrate educator-student coaching conversations.

Keywords

coachable moments
coaching questions
decision problems
decision opportunities
feedback
informal coaching
listening

Introduction

Educators in universities as subject matter experts have deep knowledge of their specialised domains and typically perform their main academic roles as instructors and academic advisors. As domain experts, many are conditioned to use a directive style of communication with students, doing a lot of "telling"

DOI: 10.4324/9781003332176-4

or "advising". Exercising restraint and not giving solutions or advice too quickly can be challenging. Students may depend on instant answers, which inhibits the development of their intellectual curiosity, self-resilience and grit. These attributes are built up gradually through determination and purposeful effort (Duckworth, 2016).

By providing immediate answers to a student's query, an educator may deprive the student of a learning opportunity by first allowing them to think independently and explore solutions. Personal growth is a continuous work in progress where learning happens through trial, error and feedback. While providing the correct answer may be quicker, it is not the most effective way to help students build a growth mindset and courage to face new challenges and attempt novel solutions (Dweck, 2017). When students develop greater intrinsic motivation, grit and self-efficacy, it helps them to become independent thinkers and confident doers.

There are many examples of different encounters with students in higher education, within and outside of scheduled timetabled hours, where coaching conversations can occur. Coaching does not always have to be a formal dialogue with prescheduled sessions. Coaching can also be short, just-in-time, informal discussions. A learning opportunity arising during and beyond formal teaching hours is a potential "coachable moment" where the educator can have a constructive dialogue with his students. University students will face "decision opportunities" that are pivotal in their educational journey. Educators can help coach students to make deliberate, value-driven decisions that can significantly impact their work and personal lives.

Coachable Moments

The concept of coachable moments originates from executive and leadership coaching literature. Turner and McCarthy (2015) define a coachable moment as:

> an informal, usually unplanned or unexpected opportunity for a manager to have a conversation with an employee aimed at facilitating the employee to problem solve or learn from a work experience. It is aimed at helping them to learn rather than instructing, directing or teaching them.
>
> (p. 5)

This description is relevant for educational institutions as well when we substitute the terms "manager" with "educator" and "employee" with "student", in the role of coach and coachee respectively. In education, a coachable moment is an opportunity to help students learn or problem-solve from day-to-day situations through reflection and discovery rather than by instructing, directing, or teaching. These situational moments are usually unplanned and informal, but the ensuing coaching conversations are timely and intentional (Lim, 2021).

Formal and Informal Coaching

Coaching does not always have to occur in formal settings, which is typical in corporate executive coaching, with hour long sessions and meetings scheduled over several weeks or months. Coaching conversations can also occur serendipitously in opportunistic situations. Grant's (2016) Quality Conversations Framework highlights that coaching conversations occur on a spectrum, from informal to formal.

Unlike formal coaching sessions based on a coaching contract with specific engagement terms, coaching in higher education settings tends to be mostly informal. Regular interactions between educators and students can yield many coachable moments. The conversation can be initiated by the educator or the student, triggered by an observation or a query. A coachable moment is invaluable as a learning opportunity because the coaching conversation can shift the student in some positive way, such as gaining clarity, attaining new knowledge and taking positive action. There are times when formal coaching sessions are necessary, such as when the student wishes to arrange a time to speak in private or when the educator asks the student to schedule a meeting on an important matter.

Essential Coaching Skills for Educators to Apply at Coachable Moments

Building rapport, developing understanding and engaging in constructive dialogue for positive coaching conversations requires good communication skills. The essential skills are:

*   Listening
*   Questioning
*   Noticing

Listening Skills

Listening is more than just hearing the other person. Active listening requires being fully present, giving full attention to the speaker and intentionally focusing on the conversation. A fully engaged educator can understand what the student is trying to convey by paying attention to the student's verbal, vocal and visual signals as a strategy for effective listening. The 3Vs are adapted from Mehrabian and Wiener's (1967) seminal research on decoding inconsistent communication. A summary of the 3Vs (verbal, visual and vocal) is shown in Table 3.1.

Table 3.1 The 3Vs Strategy for Effective Listening

3 Vs	Description
VERBAL **What is said** *The message*	• Beliefs • Humour • Interests • Language patterns • Values
VOCAL **How it is said** *Sound of the voice*	• Pitch • Rhythm • Speed • Tonality • Volume
VISUAL **What is observed** *Body language*	• Breathing • Energy level • Facial expressions • Gestures • Posture

Questioning Skills

A non-directive coaching conversation involves the educator doing mostly "asking" and very little "telling". The asking comes in the form of coaching questions. Good coaching questions are open, concise, and straightforward.

- Open questions invite the student to share more information and expand the conversation's scope. The dialogue of questions and answers can create emergent possibilities, leading to creative ideas and solutions.
- Closed questions should be avoided as they usually lead to "Yes" or "No" answers, inhibiting the conversation flow towards a richer discussion.
- Concise questions are short and easy to understand, focusing on the topic being explored. Concision can lead to smooth-flowing and meaningful dialogue.
- Straightforward questions using simple words convey the question's intent, enabling the listener to think and respond coherently. When questions are straightforward, the words can be understood. Furthermore, if the educator "stacks" questions by asking multiple questions simultaneously, it can confuse the student.

Table 3.2 summarises the questions that can be used in a coaching conversation.

Table 3.2 Asking Coaching Questions

Types of questions	Intention of questions Example of question
Analytical	**Examine causes, relationships, and pros and cons, about an issue.** • What have you contributed to this issue that you are sharing? • What is your overall assessment of the situation?
Probing	**Look at issues more thoroughly and find out details.** • Tell me what happened when you got the call. • What is the uncertainty here when you say "maybe"?
Clarifying	**Seek understanding and confirm the information being presented.** • What specifically do you mean? • How exactly do you see that happening?
Affective	**Enabling sharing of emotions and other reactions about an issue.** • How do you feel about your new work assignment? • What did you feel in your body when you finally got your answer?
Reflective	**Encourage to think deeper through introspection and prospection.** • What could you have done differently to avoid such an incident? • What lessons can you take from this to your future projects?
Connection/linkage	**Take a broader perspective by looking at relationships, and cause and effect.** • What are possible consequences of this decision on your career path? • How might other group members react to the changes you want to make?
Explorative	**Open up possibilities for exploring new ideas and gaining insights.** • Suppose … • What if …? • What else …? • What are some other options you have not considered so far?
Closing/wrap up	**Check if there is anything else before bringing the conversation to a close.** • What else would like to say before we wrap up? • Is there anything else you want to say before we end the session?

Noticing

While regular coaching conversations lead to greater proficiency and confidence, coaching can be nuanced and subtle. Raising one's coaching capabilities requires more than simply good listening and questioning skills. High emotional intelligence raises self-awareness and situational awareness, which helps an educator to develop "noticing" skills. Noticing is being observant and conscientious through non-judgmental, focused attention. A coach is more resonant and nimbler in the conversational moment with the coachee, having the acuity to sense the coachee's thoughts, emotions and behaviours (van Nieuwerburgh, 2020). For example, when coaching a student, the student may display doubt or defensiveness during the conversation. Through noticing, the educator may probe further, reframe the discussion or call out what is being noticed. The educator may share the observations with the student as feedback and be supportive to help the student reflect and find the best way forward.

Coachable Moments in a University Environment

While recognising that each student is different, they often have common issues and concerns about their educational experience. On a typical day on campus, common things you may hear students say are:

> *Prof, could you just tell me what to do? Can you please show me the solution?*
>
> *What do I need to do to get an A-grade? And why is there so little feedback given for my assignment?*
>
> *My teammate is not contributing to the project. I am doing all the work!*

These examples have the potential of being great coachable moments. Rather than give students ready solutions to their persistent questions, ask coaching questions instead. Let us explore the following student scenarios:

- Encouraging positive learning and study habits
- Supporting struggling students
- Providing feedback on academic work
- Supervising group projects.

Encouraging Positive Learning and Study Habits

For classes with regular assignments, some students are habitually late and ask for deadline extensions. Beyond abiding by the academic policy, such as deducting marks for lateness, take this opportunity for a coaching conversation. Explore with the student to explore their views about the importance of commitment to deadlines, self-accountability for academic performance and personal effectiveness. It can lead to exploring topics related to goal setting, time management and prioritisation, which are valuable skills for any university student.

Supporting Struggling Students

Underperforming and at-risk students often need more effective approaches to learning and maladaptive ways of coping with their academic workload. Students on academic warning with a low Grade Point Average (GPA) can feel demoralised and experience low self-efficacy. They may question whether they signed up for the right course or consider dropping out. When such student issues are identified early, coaching can be an excellent way to help and catch them before they disconnect from their studies, putting a brake on their spiralling problems and creating the right conditions for recovery and growth. The educator can take additional steps beyond helping them with the course content to support learning personal effectiveness skills, positive study techniques, time management and good sleep habits. More on at-risk students is covered in Chapter 6.

Providing Feedback on Academic Work

It is not uncommon to encounter students who are dissatisfied with the grades they receive for assessments. Some disgruntled students may approach the professor asking for more marks or to re-mark their assessment scripts. Others may ask for additional feedback and an explanation for the grade given even after detailed written feedback has been provided on reports returned to them. Instead of repeating the feedback already provided, educators can take a coaching approach by asking the student to review the written comments already given, followed by a conversation to clarify anything they do not understand. In addition, this can be an opportunity for a feedback and feedforward discussion, with the professor asking questions like, "What went well?", "What lessons have you learnt from this, "What would you do differently for your next assignment?" and "How can the lessons learnt here help you with your other modules?". A later section contains samples of coaching questions for feedback conversations. More detailed discussions on student feedback are covered in Chapter 5.

Supervising Group Projects

Group work and projects can have multiple learning outcomes covering technical content and other essential competencies. Conflicts amongst group members can arise, affecting task completion and quality of work. When a student complains of group disharmony, instead of immediately speaking to the accused member based on an alleged complaint, pause and consider coaching the complaining student or the collective group. This is an opportunity to help develop their emotional intelligence, communication and negotiation skills to engage difficult group members tactfully. Depending on the situation, a separate coaching conversation with the student who needs to put in more effort may be necessary. As a bonus, students can learn conflict resolution skills and improve the group's performance and grades. If the situation warrants disciplinary action against the recalcitrant student, do it after the other efforts have not been effective. For more discussion on supervising groups, see Chapter 7.

Decision to Inform a Student That They Are Being Coached

In these interactions discussed above, the student involved may or may not know they are being coached. While informing someone they are being coached sounds ideal, it may not be straightforward in some situations. Depending on the student's receptivity to coaching, some may want to get direct answers or feel defensive when informed that they will be coached. Regardless, it is possible to use a coaching approach to a conversation, whether or not the students are informed that they are being coached.

Ideally, the educator can inform all their students that they embrace coaching and use it as part of the teaching process. This helps to set expectations that sometimes, direct answers or solutions may not be provided, and coaching questions will be asked instead to nudge the students to explore and discover. For example, before meeting a student asking for additional feedback on their assignment, the educator can set the stage for the conversation by saying, "I will be using a coaching approach today. I will be inviting your contribution to the feedback conversation."

However, there are situations where an educator may not need to state that he is coaching explicitly. For example, when the educator wants to find out why this student is late for an assignment to prevent it from happening again, he may want to meet the student to discuss how the student is coping. The educator must discern whether it is best to be explicit in letting students know they are being coached. When meeting the student, they can decide if a general coaching conversation would be useful or if they need to be explicit by guiding them towards a more directed goal, such as better time management.

In other parts of the book, more practical examples of different learning contexts are discussed. This includes coaching as a group project supervisor (Chapter 7) and supporting at-risk students (Chapter 6).

Using Coachable Moments for Feedback Conversations

Coachable moments can also be used for feedback conversations. The coaching conversation can help the student to reflect on how their effort and performance has got them to where they currently are. Feedback discussions are a good springboard for a student think about future goals and action plans to achieve them.

These discussions can be a positive source of support and motivation for students. It makes them will feel appreciated, builds their confidence and inspires them to work harder. Taking the time to have these conversations makes a student feel counted as a valued individual and not just an anonymous student number in the system, which is common in large universities. Table 3.3 shows examples of coaching questions for constructive feedback conversations:

Table 3.3 Coaching Questions for Feedback Conversations

Student context	Examples of feedback coaching questions
Coachee has succeeded	• What's working well? • What are you most pleased with? • What successes have you had? • What led to this success? • What has enabled you to get this far? • Which capabilities of yours contributed to this? • Which capabilities did you grow? • What new strengths did you find? • What did you learn? • What's next for you?
Coachee has not succeeded yet	• What happened? • What challenges did you face? • How could you have dealt with those challenges? • Who may have a different perspective on what happened? • What are areas of improvement you can beef up? • What development areas would you like to work on? • What behaviours would you change for the next time? • What resources can you draw from in the future? • What will you do differently next time? • How will you move on from this?
Coachee failed or did not get started	• What happened? • What kept you from doing it? • How important is this to you? • What does this mean to you? • What will you do now? • What's next for you? • What have you learnt about yourself? • Who can you ask to help you?

Sources: Adapted from Whitmore (2017).

In Box 3.1, there is a vignette with a coaching conversation where the educator provides feedback to a student on his assessment.

The vignette illustrates that having a short coaching conversation can be powerful in encouraging reflection and creating a mindset shift. While it may take a few more conversations for the student to think beyond grades and be more learning-focused, the coaching conversation in this example was the start of a transformational journey for him. Instead of the professor doing all the work and repeating the feedback, a coaching approach can be more productive in helping the student gain insights about their performance and learn how to improve for the future, providing feedforward to move ahead and succeed. Students who want a better grade are usually driven and have high expectations for themselves, which can occasionally be unrealistic. Using powerful coaching questions can help students convert disappointment to positive energy in discovering areas for growth and potential for better performance in the future. We can use coaching questions as scaffolding support for students to reflect, become sharper and more independent in self-evaluation and identify strengths, hence building self-efficacy towards success.

Box 3.1 Providing Feedback

Augustine is a student who is highly grade orientated. He believes that it is very important to achieve excellent grades and gets very disappointed if he does not get an A. His professor, Dr M, noticed that Augustine is always asking about how he would be evaluated and what is expected for him to get the best grade.

Augustine completed a clinical oral interactive assessment, where students were assessed on their ability to respond to standardised patients' questions, integrating knowledge about developmental milestones and disabilities. Group feedback was shared with the cohort and individual feedback was provided in the learning management system. He contacted his professor wanting additional feedback as he was disappointed getting a B grade.

Dr M set the student's expectation for the meeting by informing him that she will take a coaching approach to providing additional feedback. He should be prepared to reflect and consider what he would do differently for future assessments.

At the meeting:

Dr M: Hi Augustine, I see that you would like to get additional feedback for your assessment. Before we start, tell me what you hope to achieve in the next 30 minutes of our conversation.

Augustine: Thanks for meeting me. To be honest, I am disappointed with my grade. I spent a lot of time preparing for the test and I realised that some other students who didn't seem to put in much effort fared better than me. I'm not sure why I got a B.

Dr M: I am glad to know that you have put in a lot of effort in preparing for the assessment. What would be fruitful for you to take away at the end of our meeting today?

Augustine: Hmmm … maybe you can give me more feedback on why I only got a B?

Dr M: I can guide you in discovering more about your performance and we can talk through what can be different. Let's focus on what will be most valuable for your learning. How does that sound?

Augustine: Sounds OK to me.

Dr M: Share with me how you prepared for this assessment.

Augustine: I memorised a lot of the developmental milestones. I talked to myself through the potential scenarios. I did one practice with a friend.

Dr M: From the feedback you received and your recollection, what do you think you have done well in the assessment?

Augustine: I remember I spoke a lot. So, I must have provided a lot of information.

Dr M: What else?

Augustine: I recall greeting the standardised patient professionally.

Dr M: What do you think you could improve on?

Augustine: Not sure really. I think I did pretty well.

Dr M: Let's run through part of the video recording of your assessment that day.

[Dr M played a recording of the session and paused at a few critical points. Instead of rewatching the entire assessment, she picked a salient point to pause for reflection.]

Dr M: What did you notice here?

Augustine: I spoke really fast. Kind of hard to understand.

Dr M: Indeed. I am glad you noticed. What else?

Augustine: I think I didn't really answer the patient's questions, even though I spoke a lot.

Dr M: How would you answer differently if you were to do this again?

Augustine: I would say "…."

[Dr M paused at a few points along the video and got Augustine to reflect and talk about what he would differently. She would add further comments only if he failed to identify or missed out certain observations.]

Dr M: How would you summarise your performance now?

Augustine: I think watching my video made me realise I spoke a lot but didn't answer the questions directly. I may have led my patient to be more confused. I could have slowed down and checked in if she understood me ….

Dr M: I couldn't agree more. What do you think contributed to what you just shared?

Augustine: I was very nervous as I really wanted to ace this. I thought by giving a lot of information, I could demonstrate all that I know. But now I realise it may not be helpful.

Dr M: What can you do differently in the future?

Augustine: I need to work on my nerves and slow down. Perhaps I should practise more with my friends so I can say out the answer instead of keeping it in my head.

Dr M: What else?

Augustine: Hmmm … Maybe I need to organise my thoughts better before saying them out. Then it can be less confusing.

Dr M: I am glad you picked up so many good points. Well, it is really not about the grade, but what you can learn and improve that matters. I hope this has been a useful conversation.

Augustine: Thank you! I came expecting that you would give me more feedback or consider a different grade. But now I think I can achieve more. Appreciate your time, Dr M.

Supporting Students for Decision Opportunities

Even as more mature students enrol for university courses, most undergraduates are young adults in their late teens and early 20s. Neuroscience research informs us that the human brain's prefrontal cortex, which controls decision-making and other executive functions, is fully developed when adults are in their mid-20s (Giedd, 2004). From psychology and social science research, we know that upbringing, culture, and life experience shape individual identity, values and behaviours.

Cognitive biases impact how humans think and behave. Young (2016) classifies cognitive biases into four broad categories: action-based biases, perceiving and jugging biases, framing biases and stability biases. These biases, individually and in combination, influence our perceptions and judgment of situations. Cognitive biases can lead to flawed judgements and poor decisions when evaluating choices, leading to adverse outcomes.

When educators work with students, being aware of their limitations in sensemaking and decision-making capacity due to their neurodevelopment and lived experience is helpful. It also makes the educator's role as guide, mentor and role model more critical when supporting their students in making important academic, career and life decisions.

Humans can develop greater awareness and learn skills to make good decisions. Siebert et al. (2020) summarise the essence of decision-making as our best efforts in decision-making to maximise the probabilities of making good decisions that yield positive and favourable outcomes and avoid bad decisions that result in unpleasant consequences. We face two types of decision-making situations – decision problems and decision opportunities (Keeney, 2020). Decision problems are routine decisions we make to do our daily tasks and accomplish the work we are responsible for. These ordinary and routine decisions involve alternative-focused thinking, choosing the best available options to resolve the current situation. Solving decision problems maintains or restores the decision-maker to the status quo position, with no significant shift from the previous state.

Decision opportunities are non-routine situations which require a purposeful approach to make value-based decisions (Keeney, 2020). A decision opportunity situation has the potential to achieve long-term positive outcomes, which requires more than alternative-focused thinking and not settling for default choices to maintain the status quo. The decision-maker must be proactive and deliberate in evaluating the possibilities and pathways, striving for the desired outcomes to improve the quality of life. Educators can support students with decision opportunities by helping them explore and discover beyond the familiar and impulsive choices, nudging them to reflect and examine what really matters to them, such as purpose and values, and providing guidance in the decision-making process.

An experienced educator who has gotten to know his students well over the years will know the patterns of their thinking and behaviours. This gives the educator a good entry point for coaching students thinking about their decision opportunities. Asking powerful coaching questions can help the student to stretch beyond their comfort zone to think and go deeper to explore their core values, identify strengths, and develop a future vision. Here are some examples of decision opportunities university students can encounter:

- Which subject specialisation should I choose?
- Shall I take a gap year and learn more about myself?
- Which path shall I take when I graduate ... pursue a master's degree right away or work and find a job?
- Which type of organisation should I work for upon graduation ... government, corporate sector or start-up?
- Should I work overseas to broaden my experience?
- How can I find potential jobs that are suited to my strengths?
- How will my graduation be impacted if I start a family early? (relevant for mature students)

Box 3.2 has a vignette of a coaching conversation where the educator supports his student to make the best of a decision opportunity related to career and job search.

Box 3.2   Decision Opportunities: What to Do After Graduation

The vignette is about a student's decision opportunity The coaching conversation is between a Professor and Daisy, a final year student in Computer Engineering. The meeting takes place in the Professor's office.

Professor (Prof):	Hi Daisy ... How are you? You mentioned in your email that you wanted to discuss career and jobs.
Daisy:	Hi Prof. Thanks for making the time to see me. It's my final year and I'm thinking about graduation and what kind of jobs are out there that I should apply for.
Prof:	How time flies. You will be graduating in 8 months! We have about 30 minutes today. What would you like to take away from our session?
Daisy:	I want to start working on my job search. I want a job that's interesting and can also be a stepping stone to further opportunities in the tech industry. What would you advise?
Prof:	Nice to see that you are proactive and thinking about your career. What does an ideal job look like to you?
Daisy:	Well, I am glad I chose to do Computer Engineering. I have enjoyed my university experience and love techy things and programming. I like the excitement of being in this fast-moving industry and new tech innovations excite me.

Prof: What else is important to you in finding your ideal job?

Daisy: I am a curious person and like to learn more about the latest technology. I follow the latest industry news and have attended several IT industry webinars and virtual conferences. I really aspire to be an expert.

Prof: That's great. I can feel your passion. So how can you leverage on your interests and passion in your job search?

Daisy: I can review the latest job postings on company websites. I can also do research looking at IT industry portals to see what else is out there I have not yet discovered.

Prof: OK. Tell me more about how you intend to do your research.

Daisy: I have been thinking about tech start-ups for job positions. I was reflecting on my industry attachment with a multinational corporation. I enjoyed the experience but I'm not sure working for a large company will make me happy. I feel it's more exciting working for a smaller tech start-up.

Prof: That's an interesting perspective. How much do you know about tech start-ups?

Daisy: Honestly, not very much at this stage. I would have to explore more.

Prof: What sources have you checked? Anyone you have spoken to about start-ups?

Daisy: Well, I met the career advisors at our Career Centre recently. They helped me with résumé writing and I attended seminars on job search and interview skills.

Prof: What were you able to find out from the Career Centre?

Daisy: The career advisors pointed me to various computer, engineering and infotech industry resources for job listings. However, information on start-ups was scarce.

Prof: Help me understand – explain what do you mean by scarce?

Daisy: The computer engineering and IT job listings were mainly of large multinationals and government organisations. Not much on smaller companies and tech start-ups. The Career Centre has strong connections with the larger organisations. Not so much with smaller companies and almost none in the start-up space.

Prof: Interesting. Even I did not know that. So, if you really want a job and career in the tech start-up sector, what can you do?

Daisy: That is a good question. I need think about that.

Prof: Let's look at it from a different angle. If the Career Centre, does not have the resources you need, where else can you look?

Daisy: I suppose there must be other resources from the industry and research databases of the tech start-up sector.

Prof: OK. So where will you look for more information on the tech start-up sector, if this is really your area of interest?

Daisy: Perhaps the government agencies and tech industry groups? I know the Economics Ministry publishes quarterly reports on the economy and growth sectors. From webinars and online communities I follow, I know the Startup Entrepreneurs Forum has good coverage of the start-up scene.

Prof: That's great. You have come up with some interesting ideas. What else is out there you can think of?

Daisy: I attended some industry events last year, one organised by Startup Entrepreneurs Forum and a hackathon by a tech group. I can look out for their upcoming events and also search their members directory, who are mostly start-ups.

Prof: I'm impressed that you read widely and have discovered these resources on your own. With these ideas that you have just shared, what will you do next for your job search?

Daisy: I will look out for more information these organisations have on their portals. And I will also subscribe for news updates about their management, product releases, job postings and any public events.

Prof: That is great. Besides all this, what other resources can you access for jobs?

Daisy: I am not sure …

Prof: Where do many professionals go when they are looking for jobs?

Daisy: LinkedIn … I can look at LinkedIn!

Prof: Yes, that could be a useful channel for you. How active are you on LinkedIn now?

Daisy: Not much. I have a basic profile there. Now that I am serious about my job search, especially in the tech start-up space, I will update my LinkedIn profile and be more proactive there.

Prof: Daisy, you have come up with many good ideas. After our session today, what specific action steps will take for your job search?

Daisy: First, I will look at the various online resources on the tech start-up space and identify interesting companies and job openings. Then, I will revamp my LinkedIn page and activate the alerts and other features that can help with my job search.

Prof: What else will you do?

Daisy: I will update my résumé. And upload it on selected job portals that are strong in the tech and startup space. Having a current résumé will also be handy if I apply directly to a company.

Prof:	How soon will you start?
Daisy:	I will start this weekend. I will update my LinkedIn page and review the latest postings there on evenings and weekends. I will need another week to update my résumé and then find the right job portals where I can upload it. Researching the start-up sector and tech industry will take more work … I am already monitoring this space but for an effective job search, I need to be more strategic. There is a long weekend coming up soon so that will be a good time to start on that.
Prof:	Sounds like you have an action plan and are ready to go. Is there anything else you would like to discuss today?
Daisy:	I think I have enough to work with. Nothing more for now. Thank you so much for your time. This has been a great session.
Prof:	You are welcome. All the best and keep my posted on how things are working out for you.

In this vignette, the student is thinking about what comes after graduation. Her concerns are about her career path and finding a job in her area of interest. This is a decision opportunity with consequential long-term outcomes for the student. Asking powerful coaching questions makes the coachee think and reflect on her strengths, career interests, and job preferences, and to stretch her thinking to explore opportunities beyond her comfort zone. The student is highly motivated as she wants to find a job and is willing to work hard to realise her goal. Notice that the professor did not give direct advice. The coaching relationship may not end after a single session. There could be follow-up conversations with the student sharing updates and seeking additional support from the professor as she navigates her job search journey.

Conclusion

This chapter aims to help educators identify coachable moments within the education context. We briefly shared essential coaching skills needed for a good conversation, followed by common scenarios where such coaching skills can be applied. University students face many decision-making situations in their learning journey, from first year to graduation. Educators influence and impact their students' lives through interactions with them. At appropriate moments of engagement, educators can help students to discover their beliefs, values, strengths and best hopes. These insights can help the students gain clarity, develop good judgment and navigate the pathways of their academic, career and life aspirations. In coaching conversations, asking good coaching questions serves as a nudge and scaffold that helps students make constructive decisions, leading to positive outcomes.

Discussion Starters

- What are examples of coachable moments in your interaction with students in the context of your role in your institution?
- List some coaching questions that you can use in your coaching conversations that will resonate with different types of students in various academic settings.
- When do you usually give feedback to students? How would you do it differently if you could identify coachable moments for feedback coaching conversations?
- What decision opportunities did you face as a young adult? How different do you think decision opportunities are for students in university today?

References

Duckworth, A. (2016). *Grit: The power of passion and perseverance*. Scribner.
Dweck, C. S. (2017). *Mindset - updated edition: Changing the way you think to fulfil your potential*. Robinson.
Giedd, J. N. (2004). Structural magnetic resonance imaging of the adolescent brain. *Adolescent Brain Development: Vulnerabilities and Opportunities, 1021*(1), 77–85. https://doi.org/10.1196/annals.1308.009
Grant, A. M. (2016). The third 'generation' of workplace coaching: Creating a culture of quality conversations. *Coaching: An International Journal of Theory, Research and Practice, 10*(1), 37–53. https://doi.org/10.1080/17521882.2016.1266005
Keeney, R. L. (2020). *Give yourself a nudge: Helping smart people make smarter personal and business decisions*. Cambridge University Press. https://doi.org/10.1017/9781108776707
Lim, S. M. (2021, May 27). *The answer is not always the solution: using coaching in higher education*. Times Higher Education. www.timeshighereducation.com/campus/answer-not-always-solution-using-coaching-higher-education
Mehrabian, A., & Wiener, M. (1967). Decoding of inconsistent communications. *Journal of Personality and Social Psychology, 6*(1), 109–114. https://doi.org/10.1037/h0024532
Siebert, J. U., Kunz, R. E., & Rolf, P. (2020). Effects of proactive decision making on life satisfaction. *European Journal of Operational Research, 280*(3), 1171–1187. https://doi.org/10.1016/j.ejor.2019.08.011
Turner, C., & McCarthy, G. (2015). Coachable moments: Identifying factors that influence managers to take advantage of coachable moments in day-to-day management. *International Journal of Evidence Based Coaching and Mentoring, 13*(1), 1–13.
van Nieuwerburgh, C. (2020). *An introduction to coaching skills: A practical guide* (3rd ed.). SAGE Publications.
Whitmore, J. (2017). *Coaching for performance: The principles and practice of coaching and leadership*. Nicholas Brealey Publishing.
Young, J. H. (2016). *Mindfulness-based strategic awareness training: A complete program for leaders and individuals*. John Wiley & Sons. https://doi.org/10.1002/9781118938003

4 Empathetic Coaching Conversations

Being Emotionally Present and Connected with Students

Kyrin Liong and Nadya Shaznay Patel

Chapter Objectives

- To introduce and explain the **Connect–Converse–Coach** framework as a structured approach for conducting empathetic coaching conversations.
- To provide strategies and techniques for fostering a meaningful connection and open dialogue with students.
- To address the distinction between empathetic coaching and coddling and how we can balance empathy and accountability.

Keywords

acknowledging emotions
coaching conversations
empathy
empathetic coaching
emotional connection
psychological safety

Introduction

This chapter explores Empathetic Coaching Conversations within higher education, emphasising their pivotal role in fostering strong student-educator relationships and their transformative power in guiding students towards self-discovery and growth.

The **Connect–Converse–Coach** framework is introduced as a structured approach to such conversations. This begins with building a meaningful rapport and **Connection** with students, creating a psychologically safe space for authentic and open **Conversations**. Once trust is established, educators can

DOI: 10.4324/9781003332176-5

effectively **Coach** students by demonstrating empathy for their wellbeing while holding them accountable for progress.

The chapter suggests and discusses various strategies and techniques for each framework aspect. Additionally, the chapter addresses the misconception that empathetic coaching entails coddling, underscoring the importance of balancing empathy and accountability. This chapter thus serves as a comprehensive guide for educators seeking to cultivate emotionally present and connected relationships with their students through empathetic coaching conversations.

What Are Empathetic Coaching Conversations?

Empathetic conversations, within the context of coaching and student interactions, involve our ability as educators to understand and perceive our students' feelings deeply and communicate this care through our behaviour (Meyers et al., 2019). When combined with a coaching approach, these conversations can hold up a proverbial mirror to our students, facilitating clarity in self-reflection and eventually empowering them to explore their next steps. Therefore, empathy's significance in the classroom cannot be overstated.

In education, research emphasises the crucial roles of empathetic concern and relationship-building in supporting students. Cooper (2011) underscores the significance of empathy in the classroom, stating that it contributes to creating inclusive learning environments. Regarding the integration of empathetic and dialogic interactions within classroom discourse, Patel (2023) found that students recognised these experiences when they felt "(1) cared for as individuals, (2) a sense of support in their learning, and (3) acknowledged for the struggles they faced" (p. 63). Therefore, by expressing empathetic concern, educators can effectively engage with students, fostering a more profound understanding and demonstrating care for their wellbeing. This empathetic approach is valuable in coaching conversations, as it establishes rapport and develops a trusting relationship with students.

Recognising the significance of empathetic conversations, it is essential to understand that empathy, like a muscle, can be developed and strengthened. While basic empathy is inherent in humans, trained empathy can be cultivated as a skill, particularly within professional settings (Morse et al., 1992). While individuals, especially those with atypically developed like high-functioning autism, may vary in their capacity for empathy (Baron-Cohen & Wheelwright, 2004), scholars suggest that it can be enhanced through conscious training, similar to developing professional communication skills.

However, when considering coaching conversations in an academic context, educators often believe they can only provide limited support to students, as illustrated in the following sentiment.

A coaching conversation? Moreover, it has to be empathetic? I'm not trained for this. What if I say something wrong or I make things worse?

As educators, we may instinctively experience unease when supporting students (Schneeberger McGugan et al., 2023), fearing that we might exacerbate the situation or provide inadequate guidance. Nonetheless, it is crucial to acknowledge that this unease may stem from a sincere concern for the wellbeing of our students and our desire to provide the best possible help. Hence, even if immediate desired outcomes are only sometimes attainable, we can still take a proactive approach by initiating conversations and prioritising the best interests of our students.

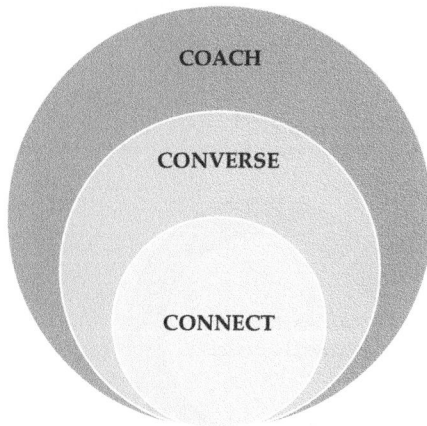

Figure 4.1 The 3Cs framework: Connect–Converse–Coach, using empathetic coaching conversations with students

To achieve this, we employ the **Connect–Converse–Coach** framework (Figure 4.1). The initial step involves establishing a **Connection** with our students, a foundation for creating a psychologically secure environment. This enables us to engage in meaningful **Conversations** grounded in trust. Once a strong connection has been formed and an open dialogue is fostered, we can effectively engage in the **Coaching** phase. A meaningful, empathetic conversation can occur in this crucial final step, aiding students' subsequent solution-focused progress.

Connect: Building a Trusting Bond

Educators must recognise that cultivating a relationship with students is essential for engaging in meaningful, empathetic coaching conversations. Thus, establishing a connection (Fuller et al., 2021) with our students is the initial and fundamental step towards facilitating effective coaching conversations.

To embark on this process, we must acknowledge that our roles extend beyond that of mere instructors. We serve as knowledgeable guides, impart valuable insights and as real-life exemplars of success within the relevant domain. Additionally, we adopt the role of a coach, offering support, encouragement and guidance throughout their academic journey (Figure 4.2).

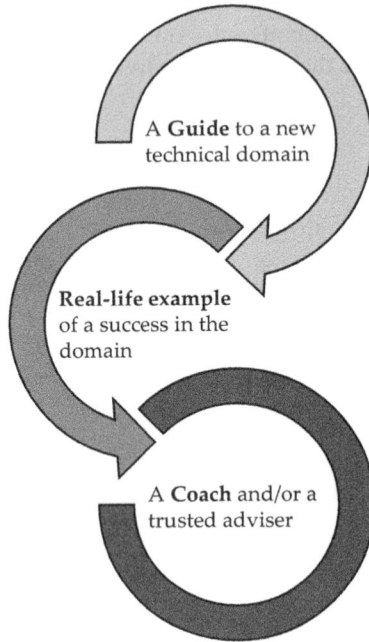

Figure 4.2 Our roles as educator

In our most obvious role as domain experts, we often find ourselves introducing students to the academic world within a technical realm. This transition can be overwhelming for school leavers who are entering a new educational environment, as well as for adult learners who are returning to education to further their skills. The curriculum's intensity and rigour can often evoke anxiety and self-doubt. Suppose we shift our perspective from being "experts" to "knowledgeable guides", we can help orient learners to this new world while openly answering their questions about navigating it successfully. In this way, we provide a comforting presence to students during this transformative period.

As guides, we also serve as real-life examples of successful professionals who have navigated the domain knowledge to build fulfilling careers. For undergraduates and sometimes adult learners, university educators may be the primary professionals with whom students spend significant time (Saphier et al., 2008). Therefore, we become the closest tangible representation of what education can achieve. This role holds significant potential for influencing the lives of our students, laying the groundwork for our ultimate role as their coaches.

As we consider the natural progression towards assuming the role of a coach, it is important to recognise the intentional and unintentional impact we may have on our students. The intentional influence is evident in the careful planning of classroom activities and the materials we use during our sessions. Unintentional influence may appear in our casual exchanges with our students. The conversations we engage in and the language we employ can profoundly impact students in unexpected ways. To illustrate this point, we invite you to read Box 4.1, which provides an account of a first-year undergraduate student named Kerry and his interactions with two professors: Joelle, who tends to express herself hastily, and Taylor, who considers his remarks more thoughtfully.

Box 4.1   Kerry's Different Experiences Interacting with His Professors

A Hasty Comment

Prof Joelle (laughs):	Oh my, that was definitely wrong.
Kerry's thought:	I said something silly. She's successful in her work; she must be right. I'm so bad at this class.

A Thoughtful Comment

Prof Taylor:	It's okay. Today's material is more difficult than others. Let's take a break and come back and talk about this later?
Kerry's thought:	Hmm, even the professor needs a break. If he has had bad moments and succeeded, then maybe I can too.

The interaction above reveals the significant impact that even minor language adjustments can have on students' learning and self-perception. Reflecting on our experiences as students, we may recall how certain remarks, deliberate or made in haste, lingered in our minds long after they were spoken. Thus, seemingly inconsequential comments during interactions can make a lasting impression and influence students' subsequent decisions (Dweck, 2017).

This serves as a reminder that, as educators and coaches, we cannot control how students internalise our words. Therefore, we must ensure our words consistently emanate from a place of empathy and kindness. By adopting a positive and empathetic approach as a coach and acknowledging that everyone faces challenges, our choice of words will follow suit, allowing us to impact our students positively. In doing so, we provide them with role models who possess expertise and demonstrate resilience in the face of difficulties. In turn, students may begin to perceive us as authentic individuals whose words carry credibility and trustworthiness (Brookefield, 2006), fostering trust between them and us. Only then will they be open to genuinely learning from and with us.

These three roles of guide, real-life success example and coach are crucial for building connections with students. By embracing these roles and employing them appropriately, we can establish early emotional connections and strengthen them by actively listening to students' concerns and fostering an environment where they feel comfortable sharing their experiences (Fuller et al., 2021). These conversations can occur in various settings, from casual exchanges to in-depth dialogues. Regardless, these interactions allow us to demonstrate care for our students and their success (Hill, 2016), laying the foundation of a trusting bond.

In the next section, we explore techniques and activities that can further deepen our initial connections with students through conversation. Whether in a large classroom or small group discussions, these approaches aim to create a safe space for engaging in empathetic coaching conversations.

Converse: Creating a Safe Space

With an early emotional connection, educators can focus on nurturing this bond to foster a psychologically safe space. This environment encourages students to ask questions openly, seek help willingly (Edmondson, 1999) and, above all, feel supported. Conversations are vital in creating such an atmosphere, making it indispensable for effective coaching.

Engaging in conversations in various settings, including informal spaces like hallways, canteens, and the more formal classroom setting, is vital for creating a safe space. Educators convey respect, interest and warmth through active listening, validating students' thoughts and feelings, and providing guidance and support (Meyers, 2011). These approaches contribute to establishing a positive rapport, leading to increased student engagement and enhanced enjoyment of the learning experience (Benson et al., 2005). Ultimately, this fosters a sense of belonging and encourages students to freely share their concerns, questions, and aspirations within this newly created safe space.

At the same time, it is essential to acknowledge that we all have finite energy, and it is prudent to direct it where it can have the most positive impact. By shifting our focus from "fixing" students to **understanding** them, educators can prioritise creating a safe space for open conversations (Demirbolat, 2006), transcending the sole emphasis on academic performance. It is worth noting that the goal is **not** to guarantee that all students will be pleased and grasp the course material quickly. Instead, the primary motivator is establishing an environment where students feel celebrated for their successes and supported in their struggles.

Nevertheless, no matter how well-intentioned, engaging in empathetic conversations with a large class of students can feel overwhelming. Educators can manage this process logistically and emotionally by adopting a strategic and incremental approach. Educators can foster an authentic and seamless rapport with students by starting early in the semester and gradually building upon these discussions throughout the term. This approach allows trust and connection to evolve naturally over time.

Students and instructors face unfamiliarity and uncertainty at the start of a new class, leading to anxiety and apprehension. To address this, instructors can establish a positive classroom tone by setting guidelines or "ground rules" and engaging students in inclusive activities promoting community and belonging. Table 4.1 provides several recommended activities to create an open, safe classroom climate and help foster this budding relationship.

Students become more comfortable with their professors as the academic year progresses, and student–faculty connections improve. In a whole class setting, instructors may ask questions tailored to individuals or smaller groups of students. These questions can include:

* "How are you feeling today?"
* "What are your thoughts on that answer?"
* "How would you approach this task?"

Table 4.1 Strategies Aimed at Creating a Safe Learning Environment for All Students, Particularly During the Initial Stages of a Course

(i) Establishing ground rules for classroom behaviour	Creating a psychologically safe classroom begins with setting agreed-upon ground rules that foster encouraging and safe conversations as a regular part of the class. Examples include: 1. We will treat ourselves and others as whole individuals, understanding that everyone has good and bad days and showing empathy instead of judgment. 2. We will try our best to adopt a growth mindset, viewing feedback as an opportunity for development rather than criticism. 3. We will try our best to realise when we have slipped into a fixed mindset and move to shift our perspective.
(ii) Encouraging regular sharing and discussion: 3-2-1 summaries	Incorporating a 3-2-1 exercise at the start or end of each class provides students with the opportunity to recall 3 key points from the previous class, share 2 standout aspects of the current week's session, and ask 1 burning question. This exercise promotes interaction among students and the faculty, highlighting that everyone experiences doubts and strengths, and that learning is a continuous journey.
(iii) Fostering laughter and team learning	Introducing simple but fun activities in the classroom can alleviate students' stress and enhance their engagement with the material. For example, engaging in popular childhood games like *Twister* or *Monopoly* can demonstrate real-life concepts such as vectors in an engineering class or financial strategies in a business class. By sharing laughter and learning through these activities, students not only enjoy the educational experience but also foster a sense of camaraderie with their peers and professor (Table 4.2). This shared humour contributes to building a positive relationship and a safe space within the classroom.

We invite you to read Box 4.2, where we return to our student Kerry and his experience of a safe classroom space.

Box 4.2   Kerry's Experience of a Safe Classroom Space

Kerry walks into class. He's initially surprised when the professor greets him, "Morning! How are you today?" He's not accustomed to professors being informal in class. He stands there as he waits for his answer, and he hesitantly replies.

Kerry:	OK, I guess. Just a bit tired.
Prof Taylor:	Oh no, why?
Kerry (thinking to himself):	He's asking follow-up questions. Goodness. I just want to sit down.
Kerry:	Just quite a few assignments and tutorials to clear Prof.
Prof Taylor:	I see. Yes, freshman year can get quite intense. [Despite his prior discomfort with the questioning, Kerry notices the professor's empathy and genuine concern for his situation. Throughout the tutorial, the professor continues to ask the class questions, causing Kerry to feel uneasy about being asked his opinion so regularly.]
Kerry (thinking to himself):	I really don't want to sound stupid. I'm going to keep quiet and let someone else answer.
Riley (Kerry's classmate):	Professor, is it because the function we're looking at reflects the previous graph?
Prof Taylor:	Hmm, what leads you to think it's a reflection, Riley?

[Kerry believes Riley's answer is incorrect but is surprised when the professor doesn't immediately correct her. Instead, he listens intently to Riley's explanation, allowing other classmates to join in on the conversation without dominating the discussion. Kerry takes note of this and observes as the professor refrains from speaking too much and instead allows the class to share their thoughts.]

Box 4.2 demonstrates how Professor Taylor's genuine interest in Kerry's wellbeing and the class's ideas create a safe space that promotes open conversation. The professor's approach of listening attentively and valuing students' perspectives rather than quickly correcting incorrect answers reinforces the sense of safety in the classroom.

We can see here how repeated similar interactions would create a positive relationship, resulting in an encouraging and engaging classroom climate. In these cases, particularly when the instructional design of the class is geared towards discussion-centred activities and sessions where there are ample opportunities for student expression and feedback, the student–faculty relationship is easily incrementally strengthened. This points to the "micro-relational components of relationship building where one small act follows another" across the semester, and their cumulative meaningfulness results in emotional engagement (Douglas & Carless, 2016, p. 212).

As we examine the intricacies of these interactions, it becomes crucial to identify the factors that contributed to Kerry's sense of safety. One vital aspect was the professor's **recognition of the value** of Kerry and his classmates' thoughts and opinions. While there are various ways to establish a positive relationship and a secure environment, specific essential strategies highlighted in Figure 4.3 are crucial when dealing with a new class of students

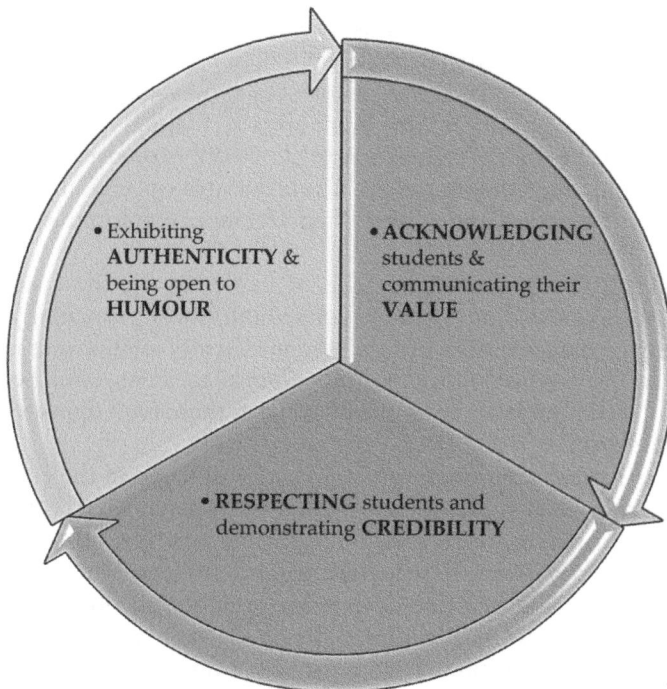

Figure 4.3 Key strategies to focus on when conversing with students

Acknowledging Students and Communicating Their Value

Acknowledging students' needs (Demirbolat, 2006), ideas and emotions will communicate that their contributions are valued and appreciated (Douglas & Carless, 2016). Furthermore, when students perceive that their professors genuinely care about them as individuals (Vuckovic et al., 2019), it fosters trust and a sense of belonging, which is essential for cultivating a safe learning environment. More crucially, when students feel secure and supported, they are more inclined to seek help and guidance from their instructor when needed.

Respecting Students and Demonstrating Credibility

Demonstrating congruence between what we say and do establishes credibility and earns students' respect (Brookefield, 2006). By honouring our commitments and following through on our words, we show respect for students and gain their trust.

Exhibiting Authenticity and Being Open to Humour

To dispel students' perceived feelings of intimidation often associated with the titles of "professor" or "lecturer", it is essential to reveal aspects of ourselves and demonstrate authenticity (Brookefield, 2006; Fuller et al., 2021). Sharing subject-related stories and personal experiences allows students to relate to us, fostering a genuine connection. This humanises us, making us more approachable and relatable to students (Vuckovic et al., 2019). Moreover, incorporating humour into our interactions creates a relaxed atmosphere, enabling better connections with students and making them feel more comfortable speaking to us when they need support.

Table 4.2 provides practical examples of implementing these strategies in the classroom. The techniques are categorised into those particularly useful at the beginning of the semester when the student–faculty relationship is new and those that can be employed throughout the term as the connection deepens. Of course, these techniques can be applied whenever there is an opportunity for a positive interaction.

With the various techniques and strategies employed in the classroom, a trusting and respectful student–faculty relationship may now be established. This connection may have significant academic benefits, but more importantly, it enables professors to recognise when a student is struggling and to initiate a coaching conversation to provide support. In other cases, where students may not outwardly exhibit signs of distress, a strong relationship can encourage them to approach their professor for help independently. The following section will explore the techniques for conducting empathetic coaching conversations.

Table 4.2 Strategies for Building Relationships through Conversation

	Beginning of the term	Throughout the term
Acknowledging students & communicating their **Value**	• Calling students by name • Making eye contact during discussion (Kolbe et al., 2020) • Welcoming them back after a break or absence (Saphier et al., 2008) • Interrupting a lesson periodically to ask for questions to check their understanding (frequently and broadly across the class) (Saphier et al., 2008)	• Asking how their day is going and listening • Incorporating their points of view into discussions (Kolbe et al., 2020) • Inquiring for details rather than making assumptions (Saphier et al., 2008) • Actively listening to them, showing interest in their ideas even when they are not fully formed
Respecting students & demonstrating **Credibility**	• Practising information transparency (Demirbolat, 2006) by openly sharing the reasoning behind the chosen learning activities and assessment tasks. • Maintaining consistency in class policies and grading (Brookefield, 2006) • Acknowledging that students will prefer certain classroom tasks and assessments over other formats, and that is why there is variety across the learning activities	• Encouraging active participation and reflection in class, and expressing appreciation for students' contributions (Kolbe et al., 2020) • Creating a supportive environment where students have the opportunity to contribute in various ways, such as through written responses or online platforms, as they gain confidence (Brookefield, 2006)
Exhibiting **Authenticity** and being open to **Humour**	• Demonstrating the ability to laugh at oneself or not taking minor hiccups in class too seriously, such as audio-visual problems or printing errors • Using humour to frame a particular concept or problem, creating a relaxed atmosphere and fostering openness to learning • Appreciating and laughing with students when they make a joke (Saphier et al., 2008)	• Periodically sharing an appropriate anecdote that relates to the concepts being taught or how we have dealt with similar struggles (Brookefield, 2006)

Coach: Empowering Self-Reflection and Growth

Having established a trusting bond through connection and a psychologically safe space through conversation with students, the next step in the **Connect–Converse–Coach** framework is to coach students through empathetic conversations. This involves intentional listening, reflecting and responding to students' needs (Noddings, 2012), aligning with the relational pedagogy approach, and emphasising care to build strong instructor–student relationships (Aspelin, 2014). Employing this approach shifts the focus of instructor–student interaction towards building an emotionally present and connected relationship rather than a dichotomous student-centred or teacher-centred approach (Patel, 2021). The effort is therefore directed at valuing and appreciating students' needs and integrating them into the coaching conversation goals (Patel, 2023).

As adopted in Patel's (2023) research on empathetic and dialogic interactions during classroom discourse, we also utilise part of the Empathic Patterns in Interpersonal Communication (EPIC) conceptual model (Weinberger et al., 2022) to facilitate empathetic coaching conversations effectively. The model identifies certain cognitive elements of empathy, including (i) positioning the conversation, (ii) employing open-heart strategies, and (iii) managing reactions. Table 4.3 briefly discusses the importance of these elements and suggests strategies for their implementation.

Table 4.3 Strategies to Model Cognitive Elements in the Empathic Patterns in Interpersonal Communication (EPIC) Model

Positioning the conversation	This element aims to establish a solid foundation for the interaction by beginning in a focused, positive, and promising manner. One simple example of achieving this is through the use of opening remarks that convey a positive spirit and trust.
Open heart strategies	To cultivate an atmosphere of empathy, these strategies call for attentive listening without prejudice, suspending judgment and engaging in a respectful dialogue that fosters opportunities for mutual learning. The emphasis should be on the other person, with speakers shifting their attention accordingly. Some examples of these strategies include: • Listening attentively (even if it is a different point of view) • Echoing the words of the other (paraphrasing) • Using expressions that acknowledge difficulties • Stepping into the shoes of the other • Encouraging dialogue by inviting a response • Asking open and clarifying questions • Using the plural forms (e.g. we), which express partnership
Managing reactions	This element seeks to create a foundation for constructive interaction by evoking mutual awareness of each other's presence, feelings of value, belonging and trust (Shady & Larson, 2010). One effective way to achieve this is by employing explanations, rationalisations, and reasoning during the conversation.

We now revisit the case of our student, Kerry, in Box 4.3, where he shares his challenges in a course with his professor. This interaction serves as an

Box 4.3   Kerry's Experience of an Empathetic Coaching Conversation with Professor Avadhani

Kerry is a student in Professor Avadhani's Critical Thinking course and has struggled to grasp some critical thinking tools used to deconstruct academic texts. Additionally, the course contextualisation within his programme in Pharmaceutical Engineering, a new field for him, further adds to the challenge. Seeking guidance, Kerry requests a discussion with Professor Avadhani.

Prof Avadhani: Hi Kerry, I am so glad to see you. I appreciate your initiative to discuss your learning. It shows excellent conscientiousness. (*Positive opening remarks*)

Kerry: Thank you, Prof.

Prof Avadhani: How do you feel when you start to read the assigned articles? (*Asking open and clarifying questions*)

Kerry: I get anxious and lost. It feels so overwhelming.

Prof Avadhani: It is natural to feel overwhelmed when practising critical reading skills more explicitly. (*Echoing the words of the other*)
I can relate to that. As a student, I also found it challenging to complete readings before lectures. (*Stepping into the shoes of the other*)

Kerry: Really, Prof? You struggled too as a student?

Prof Avadhni: Yes, I did. (*smiles*) Please tell me more about your experience.

Kerry: My main worry is that I must read the article multiple times before truly understanding it. I need to figure out where to start with the critical thinking tools or how to ask critical questions. I feel confused and lost.

Prof Avadhani (listening attentively):   I'm sorry you're experiencing these feelings, Kerry. I'm glad you shared them with me. What made you want to see me for a discussion? (*Encouraging dialogue by inviting a response*)

Kerry: Your assurance in class that you're always open for us to chat about our learning experiences encouraged me to get your advice on learning to use better the tools you taught us.

Prof Avadhani: That's great. Let's work together to explore how you can gain confidence and clarity in applying those tools. (*Using plural forms that express partnership*)

[They both reviewed a sample article on Using Animals for Testing Drugs, which the class was given for a deconstruction task, sharing their thoughts out loud as they read the article. The eventual goal is to unpack and highlight arguments made by the author using critical tools like implications, assumptions and significance.]

Prof Avadhani:	Now that we have discussed the main points, let's look at the inferences we have gained. What do you think?
Kerry:	I don't understand. Is there an assumption? And why should I consider anything beyond the author's point of view?
Prof Avadhani (smiles and listens attentively):	I understand it can be difficult to substantiate your inferences and assumptions. Would you like me to clarify the task again? (*Using expressions that acknowledge difficulties*)
Kerry:	Yes, please, Prof.
Prof Avadhani:	This task allows us to be objective about reasoning. We want to identify the flaws in this alternative claim and uncover our confirmation bias. It helps us see the flaws in the reasoning. (*Using explanations, rationalisations, and reasoning*)
Kerry:	So, we can't take the author's arguments at face value, right? That helps, actually.
Prof Avadhani:	Yes, Kerry. Well done. Let's continue. What will help you make sense of all the arguments as you step back to look at them overall?
Kerry:	I could use a concept map or arrange them in my way and place them next to the article I'm critically reading.

[Professor Avadhani smiles, nods and continues guiding Kerry with the rest of the task.]

exemplar of an empathetic coaching conversation, using the EPIC model to highlight the cognitive aspects of empathy. Through analysing this exchange, our objective is to demonstrate the profound influence of intentional empathetic coaching on our student's learning journey and its role in fostering a nurturing academic environment.

In Box 4.3, we observe the implementation of various empathy-based strategies in fostering caring instructor–student interactions. These strategies contribute to empathetic and dialogic exchanges within the classroom, making students feel valued as meaningful conversation partners with their instructor (Patel, 2023).

Moreover, this approach inspires students to reciprocate care for their instructor, leading to academic success and professional growth. As both students (the cared-for) and instructor (the carer) fulfil their roles in perceiving and delivering care, a positive and nurturing relationship is cultivated (Johnston et al., 2022).

Coaching Is Not Coddling: Misconceptions About Empathetic Coaching

Empathetic coaching revolves around understanding, compassion and support for students, but it should not be confused with coddling, which involves an overly indulgent and overprotective approach.

In this coaching method, students are encouraged to face challenges, receive constructive criticism and stretch their expertise while in an environment where high expectations and high support co-exist (Walesh, 2012). The ultimate aim is to empower students to become resilient and self-directed learners (Critchley, 2010), even if it means engaging in challenging conversations and facing discomfort to facilitate growth and development.

Hence, for empathetic coaching to be effective, it must strike a balance between empathy and accountability. This entails acknowledging students' emotions and challenges while holding them responsible for their actions and progress (Robertson et al., 2020). The process involves setting clear expectations, providing constructive feedback and encouraging students to take ownership of their learning, thus fostering personal responsibility, problem-solving skills and resilience.

However, it is crucial not to mistake accountability in empathetic coaching for punishment or blame. Instead, it involves guiding students to comprehend the consequences of their actions, learn from their mistakes, and make better decisions through open and respectful dialogue. This way, empathetic coaching achieves a delicate equilibrium, providing emotional support and encouragement while fostering student responsibility and resilience.

Conclusion

This chapter seeks to guide educators in fostering empathetic coaching conversations using the **Connect–Converse–Coach** framework. The emphasis lies in creating a psychologically safe environment where such transformative interactions occur. Kerry's story illustrates this process, from initially feeling unsafe to engaging in a coaching conversation with his professor through the EPIC model. Strategies and techniques are offered for educators to embrace this student-centred approach while finding the right balance between coaching and coddling.

Guided by genuine concern and empathy, the **Connect–Converse–Coach** framework ensures that coaching conversations go beyond surface-level interactions, leaving students with a positive impact and an impactful educational journey.

Discussion Starters

Educators can use some conversation starters and questions to implement the **Connect–Converse–Coach** framework. These prompts are designed to help educators prepare, reflect on their practice, identify areas for growth and development, and improve their support for all students:

- How can you create a classroom environment that fosters psychological safety and trust between yourself and your students?
- How might you establish and maintain an open line of communication with your students from the beginning of the course?
- How can you encourage students to share their thoughts, feelings and concerns with you non-judgementally and empathetically?
- How might you use active listening skills to understand your students' perspectives better and respond in a helpful way?
- How can you balance supporting and guiding your students and encouraging them to take responsibility for their learning and growth?
- What strategies can you use to monitor and assess the wellbeing of your students throughout the course, and how will you respond if you notice any signs of distress or struggle?
- How can you be mindful of the power dynamic between yourself and your students and work to establish a collaborative, rather than hierarchical, relationship?

References

Aspelin, J. (2014). Beyond individualised teaching: A relational construction of peda-gogical attitude. *Education Inquiry*, 5(2), 23926. https://doi.org/10.3402/edui.v5.23926

Baron-Cohen, S., & Wheelwright, S. (2004). The empathy quotient: An investigation of adults with asperger syndrome, high functioning autism, and normal sex differences. *Journal of Autism and Developmental Disorders*, 34(2), 163–175. https://doi.org/10.1023/B:JADD.0000022607.19833.00

Benson, T. A., Cohen, A. L., & Buskist, W. (2005). Rapport: Its relation to student attitudes and behaviors toward teachers and classes. *Teaching of Psychology*, 32(4), 237–239. https://doi.org/10.1207/s15328023top3204_8

Brookefield, S.D. (2006). *The skillful teacher: On technique, trust and responsiveness in the classroom* (2nd ed.). Jossey-Bass.

Cooper, B. (2011). *Empathy in education: Engagement, values and achievement.* Continuum International Publishing Group. https://doi.org/10.5040/9781472552952

Critchley, B. (2010). Relational coaching: Taking the coaching high road. *Journal of Management Development*,29(10),851–863.https://doi.org/10.1108/02621711011084187

Demirbolat, A. O. (2006). Education faculty students' tendencies and beliefs about the teacher's role in education: A case study in a Turkish university. *Teaching and Teacher Education*, 22(8), 1068–1083. https://doi.org/10.1016/j.tate.2006.04.020

Douglas, K., & Carless, D. (2016). My eyes got a bit watery there: Using stories to explore emotions in coaching research and practice for injured, sick and wounded military personnel. *Sports Coaching Review*, 6(2), 197–215. https://doi.org/10.1080/21640629.2016.1163314

Dweck, C. S. (2017). *Mindset – updated edition: Changing the way you think to fulfil your potential.* Robinson.

Edmondson, A. (1999). Psychological safety and learning behavior in work teams. *Administrative Science Quarterly, 44*(2), 350–383. https://doi.org/10.2307/2666999

Fuller, M., Kamans, E., van Vuuren, M., Wolfensberger, M., & de Jong, M. D. T. (2021). Conceptualizing empathy competence: A professional communication perspective. *Journal of Business and Technical Communication, 35*(3), 333–368. https://doi.org/10.1177/10506519211001125

Hill, P. (2016). Insights into the nature and role of listening in the creation of a co-constructive coaching dialogue: A phenomenological study. *International Journal of Evidence Based Coaching & Mentoring, 10*, 29–44.

Johnston, O., Wildy, H., & Shand, J. (2022). 'That teacher really likes me' - Student-teacher interactions that initiate teacher expectation effects by developing caring relationships. *Learning and Instruction, 80*, 101580. https://doi.org/10.1016/j.learninstruc.2022.101580

Kolbe, M., Eppich, W., Rudolph, J., Meguerdichian, M., Catena, H., Cripps, A., Grant, V., & Cheng, A. (2020). Managing psychological safety in debriefings: A dynamic balancing act. *BMJ Simulation & Technology Enhanced Learning, 6*(3), 164–171. https://doi.org/10.1136/bmjstel-2019-000470

Meyers, S., Rowell, K., Wells, M., & Smith, B. C. (2019). Teacher empathy: A model of empathy for teaching for student success. *College Teaching, 67*(3), 160–168. https://doi.org/10.1080/87567555.2019.1579699

Meyers, S. A. (2011). Do your students care whether you care about them? *College Teaching, 57*(4), 205–210. https://doi.org/10.1080/87567550903218620

Morse, J. M., Bottorff, J., Anderson, G., O'Brien, B., & Solberg, S. (1992). Beyond empathy: Expanding expressions of caring. *Journal of Advanced Nursing, 17*(7), 809–821. https://doi.org/10.1111/j.1365-2648.1992.tb02002.x

Noddings, N. (2012). The caring relation in teaching. *Oxford Review of Education, 38*(6), 771–781. https://doi.org/10.1080/03054985.2012.745047

Patel, N. S. (2021). Establishing social presence for an engaging online teaching and learning experience. *International Journal of TESOL Studies, 3*(1), 161–177. https://doi.org/10.46451/ijts.2021.03.04

Patel, N. S. (2023). Empathetic and dialogic interactions: Modelling intellectual empathy and communicating care. *International Journal of TESOL Studies, 5*(3), 51–70. https://doi.org/10.58304/ijts.20230305

Robertson, D. A., Padesky, L. B., Ford-Connors, E., & Paratore, J. R. (2020). What does it mean to say coaching is relational? *Journal of Literacy Research, 52*(1), 55–78. https://doi.org/10.1177/1086296X19896632

Saphier, J., Haley-Speca, M. A., Gower, R. R. (2008). *The skillful teacher: Building your teaching skills*. Research for Better Teaching, Inc.

Schneeberger McGugan, K., Horn, I. S., Garner, B., & Marshall, S. A. (2023). "Even when it was hard, you pushed us to improve": Emotions and teacher learning in coaching conversations. *Teaching and Teacher Education, 121*, 103934. https://doi.org/10.1016/j.tate.2022.103934

Shady, S. L. H., & Larson, M. (2010). Tolerance, empathy, or inclusion? Insights from Martin Buber. *Educational Theory, 60*(1), 81–96. https://doi.org/10.1111/j.1741-5446.2010.00347.x

Vuckovic, M., Riley, J. B., & Floyd, B. (2019). The first year colloquium: Creating a safe space for students to flourish. *Journal of the Scholarship of Teaching and Learning, 19*(2), 172–186. https://doi.org/10.14434/josotl.v19i1.23517

Walesh, S. G. (2012). Developing relationships. In *Engineering your future: The professional practice of engineering* (3rd ed., pp. 123–166). John Wiley & Sons. https://doi.org/10.1002/9781118160459.ch4

Weinberger, Y., Levi-Keren, M., Landler-Pardo, G., & Elyashiv, R. A. (2022). Empathic patterns in complex discourse. *Journal of Organizational Psychology, 22*(1). https://doi.org/10.33423/jop.v22i1.5109

Part II

Coaching for Academic Performance

5 Coaching Dialogue as Feedback to Improve Performance

Mara McAdams, May Sok Mui Lim and Nadya Shaznay Patel

Chapter Objectives

- To highlight the crucial role of effective feedback in facilitating holistic student development and fostering habits of self-regulated lifelong learning.
- To identify and explore the critical components of effective feedback in higher education.
- To elucidate the coaching approach to feedback, emphasising its dialogic nature, solutions-focused perspective and strengths-based orientation.
- To delve into the significance of emotional awareness and self-regulation in giving and receiving feedback and underscore the impact of leveraging positivity through a strengths-based feedback approach.
- To shed light on common challenges educators encounter during feedback dialogues and propose effective strategies to address them.

Keywords

coaching mindset
coaching approach
feedback
growth mindset
self-assessment
self-regulation
strengths

Introduction

Effective feedback, delivered thoughtfully and strategically, can catalyse transformative learning experiences in higher education. The potency of feedback dialogues can be further amplified when educators adopt a coaching approach,

DOI: 10.4324/9781003332176-7

transforming these interactions into pivotal coachable moments. This chapter is designed to guide educators in reframing traditional one-way feedback dissemination into dynamic coaching dialogues that prompt learners to recognise gaps, devise new strategies to address their learning needs, set informed goals and assert control over their learning trajectory. We will explore factors influencing effective feedback dialogues, elucidating its key features, and presenting practical strategies to manage and harness the emotional aspects intrinsic to the feedback process during coaching conversations. Hence, the coaching approach to feedback is integral to our exploration, which positions students as the drivers of change while placing educators as facilitators. By explicitly applying coaching skills and techniques, educators can empower students to derive meaningful insights from their feedback, subsequently driving the changes necessary to elevate their academic performance. This chapter is underpinned by an emphasis on holistic learner development, reflecting the principles of self-regulated learning and reinforcing the long-term potential of a coaching approach to feedback. By the end of this chapter, educators should be equipped with the knowledge and strategies to create feedback dialogues that resonate with learners and stimulate their drive for continuous learning and growth. We will begin with the narrative of a student who was frustrated with the feedback he received in Box 5.1.

Box 5.1 Introducing Gilbert

Gilbert is a third-year university student who has submitted a draft of his research paper to his lecturer for feedback. The paper lacks the organisation that Dr Tan taught in class and his citations don't follow the format taught either. As Dr Tan starts to write comments on the paper, she feels a bit of déjà vu. She looks back at her notes on the paper Gilbert submitted for the last assignment and sees the same feedback Dr Tan is now writing. She wonders, why isn't he putting my feedback into action?

Gilbert reports that he feels anxious every time he reads feedback from his instructors; he doesn't really remember what they said, just that he was worried he would get a bad mark. Gilbert shares that he doesn't intend to ignore his instructors' feedback. It is just that his anxieties make it too difficult to hear the feedback.

Gilbert doesn't feel like he is learning nor is he applying the feedback to his other written assignments. Gilbert says usually the instructor will tell him how to improve it, and he just does what he is told for the revision. He isn't learning but rather 'performing'. Gilbert doesn't see his progress holistically but just one class – and even one assignment – at a time.

Gilbert sees his instructor as having all the power. He wants to "give the instructor what she is asking for" rather than reflect on how the feedback can be applied more generally to make him a better writer. He views feedback as criticism that merely points out his flaws. He rushes through the feedback and the sense of inadequacy it generates, as quickly as possible to get back to feeling that he is capable. His anxiety and defensiveness stop him from taking in the feedback. If Gilbert continues to go through his course this way, he won't develop his knowledge and skills. He will go from assignment to assignment trying to give each instructor "what they want".

Chapter 3 explored various examples of coachable moments in higher education. One of the pivotal coachable moments is providing feedback to students so they can learn and grow. While the feedback may be related to the content of the academic subject, the process of receiving, reflecting on, and implementing the feedback develops the student holistically. Receiving feedback and applying it is an essential part of self-directed learning.

A coaching approach to feedback requires a coaching mindset (Dhawan, 2021). First, educators ask the recipient of the feedback to be proactive in the process rather than passively waiting to be told what to do differently. The coaching approach to feedback is a two-way dialogue in which the student's input is central. Second, as discussed in Chapter 2, a coaching mindset requires educators to see individuals as resourceful and have the potential to change and grow. Even if students appear disinterested or unmotivated, or if they have significantly underperformed, they have the potential to improve. Third, drawing on the solution-focused principles of "doing more of what is working", the coaching approach to feedback should always involve identifying strengths (the natural skills and abilities that individuals possess and are particularly good at) and what students have done well so that they can recognise and build on them.

Before learning more about using a coaching approach to feedback, it is important to understand some fundamentals of effective feedback.

Giving Effective Feedback

Most educators learn how to give effective feedback in school or faculty development programmes. Despite this training, educators often admit that providing student feedback remains challenging (Paris, 2022). They are right; giving effective feedback is challenging, yet educators can develop these skills through training. Giving effective feedback requires the skills of observation, clear communication and emotional intelligence. Giving feedback is more than a cognitive act. It is an emotional interaction that can challenge a student's self-view, create an uncomfortable feeling of being judged and compound fears about grades and marks. For feedback to be effective, educators must optimise the cognitive elements and manage the emotional parts of the process. This chapter will first address the cognitive aspects and, subsequently, the emotional aspects of giving effective feedback.

Originally, feedback was defined as the information educators gave to students. Now, most researchers and educators agree that feedback is how students receive performance information, reflect on it, and make improvements. Numerous studies have validated the cognitive elements that make the process effective – or "good (Jackel et al., 2017; Lipnevich & Panadero, 2021; Orsmond et al., 2011). First, good feedback is based on direct observation and focuses on modifiable behaviours rather than personal traits or styles. Second, it is specific and timely. Educators point to examples, describe the behaviour in detail and share the observations as soon as possible. Third, good feedback is given in a respectful, non-judgemental way. Educators are responsible for considering the setting, providing privacy and choosing polite and professional words and phrases. Next, effective feedback includes suggestions for improving the behaviour or using a strength better. Effective feedback does not only aim to correct past performance. It looks to improve future performance. This future-focused feedback is often referred to as "feedforward" (Sadler et al., 2022). Last, effective feedback is best conveyed to the student during a dialogue that allows for questions, clarifications and a better understanding of the motivations behind a choice or decision. For example, when feedback must be given as unidirectional comments on a submitted assignment, apply the first four guidelines above.

Unfortunately, educators often fail to apply the four cognitive elements, resulting in ineffective – or unhelpful – feedback. When feedback is not timely, students struggle to recall what was done and why. Ineffective feedback can feel like an information dump to the student or an attack on their personal traits. Critical feedback that is given publicly in a way that causes the student to feel shame or humiliation undermines the message. Students *can* learn from ineffective feedback, but the higher cognitive load and the negative emotional burden it creates makes it difficult to grasp the learning.

Coaching Approach to Feedback

The coaching approach to feedback is inquiry-based and meets the students where they are (Seko & Lau, 2021). Rather than seeing feedback as external or judgemental, this approach presents feedback as data that the student can use – or not use – for further development and learning opportunities. The coach helps guide the student to consider what the feedback means, its significance and relevance, and how addressing it would benefit the students' overall learning and progress. Through the coaching dialogue, educators support students as they work towards the desired future they have envisioned. In this way, the coaching approach to feedback embraces the concept of feedforwarding.

In good coaching conversations, educators frame their questions appropriately and tailor their feedback to the specific student at this specific moment to identify opportunities for them to reflect more deeply. For example, educators can start the coaching dialogue with open questions about students' perceptions of their performance. Here, educators can learn more about students' struggles and possible misconceptions. Next, it will be appropriate for educators to help guide students in defining their learning goals. Students must focus on specific areas of process improvement instead of merely increasing marks. Finally, educators and students can jointly create specific, feedback-informed actions to reach the goals.

The coaching approach to feedback sees students as whole and capable of directing their learning and applying the feedback they receive. It is a student-centred approach and aims to empower students to take charge of their learning. This approach flattens the hierarchy between the student and the educator (Seko & Lau, 2021). Educators are relieved of feeling that they have to "fix" the students' problems; students become accountable for addressing the feedback received.

Empowering students in this way supports the development of the self-regulation and self-management necessary to become self-directed, lifelong learners. Participation in these coaching dialogues to improve performance will encourage students to have greater trust and confidence in receiving feedback. This approach creates an alliance between educators and students. Over time, the positive feedback experiences will motivate students to seek out, reflect on and apply feedback more readily. By habituating students to be proactive in seeking feedback, reflective when reviewing their performance, and receptive and accountable to feedback received, educators prepare students for long-term career development. A further benefit of students learning these feedback skills is that they may apply them to *give* good feedback to their peers, instructors and future co-workers.

Recognising and Acknowledging Emotions during Coaching for Feedback

Emotions positively and negatively impact learning (Tyng et al., 2017). The coaching approach to feedback acknowledges the role of emotions in feedback and helps students manage their emotions to facilitate learning. In addition, feedback dialogues are an emotional experience for many students *and* educators. Educators feel anxious about giving feedback to students, while students feel anxious about getting feedback. However, in the educator–student relationship, the power dynamic favours the educator, and it is the role of the educator to take the lead on managing emotions.

The educator is often older, more experienced and the subject-matter expert. Educators mark assignments and award grades, ultimately affecting students' progression. Students want to perform well and make good grades. They apply this pressure to themselves, and many also feel pressure from their families. Whereas an educator may see suggestions for improvements as a teaching moment, some students may see these as an evaluation of their ability and self-worth. This is especially so in some cultures and education systems, which place the highest value on academic outcomes, causing students to relate grades to an assessment of their value and identity as a student (Crocker & Luhtanen, 2003). As such, even well-intentioned and well-delivered feedback can create an identity crisis for a student. It is no wonder students approach feedback with trepidation. It is challenging to listen and learn in an anxious state. Educators can help students manage their emotions by asking how they feel, acknowledging their feelings and showing empathy (Lieberman et al., 2007). (For more on empathy in coaching, see Chapter 4.) Once students have self-regulated their emotions, they are more ready to receive feedback.

While many students see feedback as an identity threat, the research on growth mindset shows that students who adopt a growth mindset about feedback see feedback as an opportunity to improve and grow (Dweck, 2006). In a growth mindset, feedback signals that "they are not there yet", and this new formative performance data will help them get there. The research into mindset shows that students can actively and deliberately shift into a growth mindset from fixed by setting the intention to see the feedback as data for them to use as they see fit. Feedback is not an evaluation of them as individuals but information with suggestions for improvement. Even in summative assessments, the feedback can be used for formative development.

Educators must also manage their emotions to create a successful feedback dialogue. Educators often feel anxious in the lead-up to a feedback conversation as they worry over the uncertainty of the student's response or have doubts about their ability to manage the emotions that may arise. Some educators worry that the feedback session may turn into a dispute over grades and marking criteria. This anxiety may cause the educator to avoid feedback conversations, leading to a lack of timeliness and loss of learning. This may lead to further self-criticism and negative emotions for the educator.

There are a few practical suggestions to help educators manage their emotions to approach feedback dialogues with more energy, optimism and positive feelings. First, educators can recognise that thoughts about how the student will respond are just thoughts, not truth. The student may be grateful for the feedback, having sensed the same thing himself, or that may be reassured that you are available to help him identify and address gaps. Suppose an educator is concerned about a student experiencing significant distress from feedback. In that case, they can invite someone from the department to join the meeting, and they can be prepared to share information about the resources the institution offers students in distress. The final suggestion is a quick reset for any anxious thoughts. Educators can name their emotion(s) and slowly exhale a deeper breath. The emotion naming and prolonged exhale trigger the parasympathetic nervous system, telling the body to relax. (Educators can suggest this technique to an anxious student as well.)

Cognitive and emotional self-regulation by students is critical for effective feedback, and the coaching approach can support this self-regulation in a few ways. Literature shows it is beneficial for students to conduct a self-assessment of their performance and to share that assessment with the educator as a starting point for the feedback dialogue (Boud & Molloy, 2012). Such self-assessment does two things. It highlights the student's level of insight into the strengths and growth areas and can help the educator understand how open to feedback the student is. As students may need time to overcome the negativity bias and acknowledge the good parts of their work, educators must ask them to identify what they did correctly to balance their self-assessment and promote self-efficacy. Questions about their feelings allow the students to become more self-aware of their emotional responses, increase emotional literacy and share their feelings openly. Once the feelings are named, educators can normalise how giving and receiving feedback is emotionally challenging. Educators can activate positive emotions by asking questions about areas they are proud of and challenges they have overcome.

Harnessing Positivity: The Strengths-Based Feedback Approach

Students' strengths and the positive aspects of their work are often overlooked or considered obvious by educators. The human brain has a negativity bias that causes us to notice and remember the bad much more readily than the good (Rozin & Royzman, 2001). Without deliberate effort, educators may not see the good in an assignment. As a result, feedback can be skewed to negative, albeit constructive, feedback. When educators are solution-focused, they see individuals as resourceful and having growth potential (Jackson & McKergow, 2007); from this lens, educators look for strengths and past successful experience (what solution-focused coaches refer to as "resourceful past") from which to draw motivation.

A strengths-based approach to feedback differs from how many educators were taught to use positives in feedback dialogues. While many educators were trained in the "feedback sandwich" method in which negative feedback is presented between two positive comments, many are moving away from this approach because feedback recipients may see the positive as merely a delay before the critical "meat" of the feedback. With the "feedback sandwich", students are often emotionally bracing themselves for the criticism to come. Sometimes, students further complicate educators' efforts at identifying and giving feedback on the positive by discrediting the positive as flattery or as a contrived buffer for the critical feedback that will follow.

In solutions-focused coaching, the goal or solution is defined by the student who is coached to identify strengths and resources to help reach the goal. Positive psychology validates strengths-based approaches as more motivating, and working from strengths rather than weaknesses helps create self-efficacy and confidence in the student (Linley et al., 2010). Looking for students' strengths, giving specific feedback on those strengths in action and encouraging students to think about ways to use the strengths further would amplify the educational impact of the feedback. (See Chapter 6 for more details on using a strengths-based approach to coaching.)

Integrating the Pieces: Towards a Solutions-Focused Feedback Coaching Paradigm

Solutions-Focused Feedback Coaching is a framework that incorporates all the evidence-based feedback recommendations into a Solutions-Focused Coaching approach (Box 5.2). It addresses all the critical issues discussed in this chapter thus far: a dialogue between educator and student, awareness and management of the cognitive *and* emotional elements of feedback, the

---

Box 5.2   Solutions-Focused Feedback Coaching

Adapted from R2C2 Feedback Model (Sargeant et al., 2016).

Relationship Building and Setting the Stage

- Build rapport and trust by asking questions and listening
- Explain that this coaching dialogue may differ from past experiences
- Emphasise that the student has the skills to create the solution
- Understand the student's context and ask for a self-assessment

Exploring Reactions to the Feedback – Cognitive and Emotional

- Share feedback, including positive feedback (strengths)
- Explore reactions, thoughts, feelings
- Acknowledge the student's responses, name the emotions that promote self-regulation
- Express empathy

Exploring Understanding and Support Meaning-Making

- Ask questions to clarify students' understanding of the feedback provided
- Explore the impact of this new data on previous learning and beliefs
- Explore how it would be helpful to apply this feedback to future assignments
- Encourage the student to ask questions to understand the feedback

Coaching for Performance Change via Goal Setting

- The miracle question can be used to envision the desired future
- Ask students to set an achievable goal by describing the steps
- Explore resources required and remind students of existing strengths
- Ask about obstacles, past attempts
- Use a scale to help students situate themselves in the present and look towards a preferred and measurable future

---

importance of guided self-assessment, and the use of coaching to empower students in their goal setting for learning. This framework is adapted from the R2C2 Facilitated Feedback Model initially developed for medical education. R2C2 is an easy-to-use, research-validated tool to guide feedback dialogues and effectively optimise student learning from feedback (Sargeant et al., 2016). Its four phases address (i) rapport and relationship building, (ii) exploring reactions to feedback, (iii) exploring feedback content and (iv) coaching for change. The Solutions-Focused Feedback Coaching framework adds a solutions-focused approach to the original R2C2 to empower students emotionally, cognitively and behaviourally to build solutions through feedback.

Common Challenges for Educators

From experience and conversations with educators, there are four common challenges when using the coaching approach for feedback. Students whom educators perceive:

- As being used to be spoon-fed
- To be defensive and challenging
- To be quiet and hesitant to contribute to the feedback dialogue
- To be asking for more marks

Students Whom Educators Perceive as Being Used to be Spoon-Fed

Educators must remember that students' attitudes towards learning and receiving feedback have been shaped by their previous learning experiences. Some education systems emphasise that there is only one correct answer or that the "instructor is always right". Alternatively, students may have found that whenever they struggle or say, "I don't know", the answer is quickly handed over, releasing them from the struggle. To address this, it helps the educator to set the expectation that feedback will be an active dialogue and then ensure it is by asking for the students' opinions, reflections and learnings. Instead of immediately accepting "I don't know" as a response, encourage the student to provide a "best guess" or suggest what they can do to find out what they do not know. The larger aim is to train the student to become a self-directed learner, and this process takes time. To promote dialogue, educators may validate and encourage responses, whether or not the responses are what the educator hoped to hear.

Students Whom Educators Perceive to Be Defensive and Challenging

Quite commonly, students who are constant achievers can be very critical and disappointed when they receive negative feedback or a grade below their expectations. While they may not know it, they often have a fixed mindset, associating success and self-worth with the grade they are receiving.

Many high-achieving students may be perfectionistic, and their self-expectations are high and unrealistic, allowing no room for mistakes or learning through errors. As a result, they reject feedback to protect their identity as a good student. In addition, critical but well-meaning family members may reprimand students for not performing well. Therefore, students may erect walls when an educator offers critical feedback. To counter this, educators can remind students that the feedback is data and not a reflection of them as a person. Educators can steer the conversation towards a preferred future of improved performance rather than a troubled past of work poorly done. It may be helpful to share a sample of past students' work (with pre-sought permission) to create a small distance for such a student, as they can be less defensive when critiquing others' work. This helps to demonstrate that mistakes are part of learning and that one's attitude toward learning defines one's ability. Following that, the educator can return to reviewing the student's work and praising the student's willingness to talk about areas of growth.

Students Whom Educators Perceive to be Quiet and Hesitant to Contribute to the Feedback Dialogue

Not all students are fast thinkers who can respond to questions about learning, motivation and decisions on the spot. Also, many students are quiet, introverted or intimidated by the educator's rank. Educators may get uncomfortable with silence, feel annoyed or even conclude that students are "waiting to be told an answer" or "unhappy about feedback". In response to this emotional discomfort, the educator might rush in to provide a hint, a prompt or an answer. That further delays the student's response and shifts focus to the educator's priorities. It may also reinforce the practice of waiting until the educator spoon-feeds the answer.

To address this challenge, signpost feedback sessions in advance and ask students to prepare a self-assessment that includes positive and negative aspects to discuss. Observe for signs of fatigue or distress. It is hard to be coached on an empty tank. If a student does not seem to be in the best frame of mind to receive feedback, share that observation and arrange for another time to meet. If the student is quiet and cannot be coached as they lack the content knowledge, it may be necessary to send the student back to learn more or use the remaining time to switch into a teaching role to fill the knowledge gaps.

Students Whom Educators Perceive to Be Asking for More Marks

Educators may also unknowingly build a self-protective wall with students who seem to be challenging them for more marks. Sometimes, students feel dissatisfied with their grades and plan to dispute a grade. Educators can turn those conversations from "seeking more marks" to "getting feedback for growth". In such instances, educators may feel they need to justify the grade and become defensive, unintentionally highlighting all the critical feedback to justify the grade decision. Worse, they may emphasise what a student must do "or else" – they will not get an A grade or they would not pass, etc. This triggers the student to take a defensive position, encoding the feedback with a survival response. Such feedback increases defences, lowers confidence, and decreases initiative and innovation (Reynolds, 2020).

To address this challenge, educators must watch their thoughts and emotions, stay neutral, and coach students to identify positive and critical feedback to help future work. What is most dangerous to the educator–student relationship is when an educator sees the student *as a problem* rather than someone *having a problem* with some aspect of their learning. The coaching approach to feedback addresses these fears by providing a clear pathway to shifting into a dialogue in which the student is responsible for their learning.

Box 5.3 is an example of such a coaching dialogue using a solutions-focused approach.

Box 5.3   Coaching Dialogue Using a Solutions-Focused Feedback Coaching Approach

Mary made an appointment to see her professor, hoping to see if she can improve her grade for the recent assignment.

Mary: I am not sure why I only received a C for the recent assignment. With my effort, it should have been an A. The written feedback is too brief, and I hope to discuss more.

Prof J: Thanks for making the arrangements to meet me today. I am looking forward to talking with you about your learning. What do you like about the course so far? *(Ask for positives, build rapport)*

Mary: I like the classroom discussions and your lectures. I like thinking through my ideas out loud and hearing other students' views. I guess I also like the topic. As a science student, I haven't taken a course in Humanities before.

Prof J: That is awesome. You frequently contribute to class and bring great ideas. And it's brave of you to choose a course in a new area of study. *(Validate positive contributions and positive self-view.)*

Mary: Well, I try my best. Glad that you do notice.

Prof J: Now, I want to talk about the feedback I provided on your paper. Is that OK? *(Set agenda, invite participation and prepare the student)* I will use a coaching approach for feedback, and I invite you to be an active part of this conversation. I won't be telling you how exactly to do things but guiding you as you interpret the feedback you received. *(Set the stage and set expectations) This* may be a different approach to feedback than you are used to. What do you think about this so far? *(Check for understanding and reactions)*

Mary: Sounds OK, but I am bit unsure. It is new to me. Can you tell me why I only got a C?

Prof J: Yes, I get it. It can be a bit scary to discuss feedback about assignments. *(Acknowledge and normalise emotions)* I am giving you this feedback because I am invested in your learning and want you to be as successful as you can be. Keep in mind that this feedback is yours to use to grow and develop. OK? *(Set the intention and activate growth mindset) What* were the strongest parts of your paper? *(As for self-assessment, highlight strengths)*

Mary: I thought I laid out my argument in the intro and then stated my case and finished with more arguments in its defence. The overall structure was quite clear.

Prof J: I agree with most of that. I liked how you …

[Prof goes on to give the positive feedback on the structure and the choice of thesis. He holds his critical feedback on adding new arguments into the conclusion until later in this dialogue.]

Prof J: Where do you think you can do better? *(Ask for self-assessment of areas of growth)*

Mary: I saw your comment about not putting new arguments in the conclusion and I get it. In fact, other instructors have been told me that before. I had more good points to make though; so I added them.

Prof J: It is great that you are connecting this feedback to past feedback and learning. Tell me more about that. *(Make connections to past experience, use open-ended questions to prompt deeper exploration)*

[Prof goes on to share the rest of the critical feedback that impacted the grade, asking Mary to suggest what changes she would make if she was to reattempt the writing.]

Prof J: How are feeling about all of this so far? *(Address emotional aspects of feedback)*

Mary: I still think I am better than a C.

Prof J: The paper got a C; you are a person who can't be graded. What can you tell yourself to shift towards a growth mindset and see this paper and its C as an opportunity? *(Acknowledge impact of mindset and student taking on the performance as a sign of self-worth, Encourage growth mindset)*

Mary: I am in a new area of study; I am out of my comfort zone. You have pointed out a bunch of areas where I didn't meet the mark for an A. I guess I can use this to get ready for the final paper that is due next month.

Prof J: Great insights …

[Prof goes on to coach her on applying the learning to other areas: How will you apply what you are learning to the other assignment? How might you apply it to other contexts? What would become possible if you applied this feedback? What is holding you back? What is the next step? What challenges do you expect? What resources do you need? The student participates in the coaching process and sets a goal of submitting a draft to her group mate for peer feedback; she will meet the word limit and keep all her arguments in the essay body.]

Prof J: How does this all seem to you? *(Check for questions and understanding)*

Mary: This process feels different, because usually profs just tell me what is wrong and all the things I should have done. Then, I have no idea what to bring forward to my next assignment. Well, this conversation was harder than being told what to do but now I have a better plan, and I can be ready to do better on the next one. I feel more confident for the final paper.

The case demonstrates that students often expect educators to tell them how to fix the problem, and educators frequently do just that. Learners in higher education need to take control of their learning to become self-directed life-long learners. Using a coaching approach for feedback facilitates that transformation by presenting feedback as data that the student can use to further knowledge and understanding. The educator coaches the learner through the process, refocusing the discussion on creating solutions, activating strengths and encouraging self-regulation of emotions, thoughts and behaviours. Box 5.4 suggests some coaching conversation starters and questions to use when giving students feedback.

Box 5.4   Coaching Conversation Starters and Questions

Coaching conversation Starters and Questions to Consider Using:

Set the Intention and Expectations

- I am giving you this feedback because I am invested in your growth and want you to be as successful as possible. Set your intention to see this conversation as data that is yours to use to grow and develop.
- Today, we will use a coaching approach for feedback, and you are invited to be part of this active process. I will not give you answers but guide you as you interpret the feedback data you receive.

Build Relationships and Acknowledge Emotions

- How are things going for you in the course?
- What did you think of this assignment?
- Getting feedback from your instructor can be scary/challenging/intimidating. That feeling is normal.

Ask for Self-Assessment

- Helping students self-assess their performance encourages ownership of their work and reflection.
- How do you feel about this piece of work?
- What is the most vital part of this work?
- What would you do differently if you were given a chance?
- What surprised you the most?
- How is hearing this feedback difficult for you?

Provide Feedback

- Of the feedback that I have shared, which are the ones that resonate with you?
- What can you tell yourself to shift towards a growth mindset and see this feedback as an opportunity?
- Please summarise the feedback that I have shared.

Coaching for Improvement

- What questions do you have?
- What are you learning about your work on this assignment?
- How can you apply this learning to other contexts?
- What would become possible if you applied this feedback?
- What is the next step?
- What challenges do you expect?
- What resources do you need, and which do you have?

Support the Student's Strengths / Agency

- You can make these changes / apply this feedback.
- It will take effort and time, but you will get there. Please contact me if you want to discuss how it is going.

Conclusion

Feedback, when employed effectively, holds the power to illuminate blind spots and stimulate profound learning opportunities. However, it often challenges educators due to various factors, such as emotional engagement and the ability to manage dialogues effectively. Acknowledging and normalising the emotions that arise during feedback conversations is a significant step towards improved self-regulation, contributing to a more efficient and meaningful feedback process. Feedback also thrives best as a two-way dialogue, commencing with the learner's self-assessment. This gives educators a deeper understanding of the learner's perception of their performance, paving the way for a more personalised, effective feedback process. The coaching approach to feedback may initially appear foreign to learners accustomed to directive types of feedback. Educators should be explicit about this process, reinforcing the importance of learner autonomy and resisting the urge to solve problems for the learners.

Students' mindset plays a pivotal role in their receptivity to feedback. Activating a growth mindset enables learners to perceive feedback as a data-driven avenue for improvement rather than a global judgement of their abilities. To counteract the brain's innate negativity bias and bolster intrinsic motivation, it is crucial to highlight strengths and positive aspects of performance. Such an approach highlights areas of success and encourages learners to leverage these strengths in areas requiring improvement. Moreover, educators and students should collaborate to set achievable goals that enhance performance. This facilitates a solution-focused approach, allowing learners to draw from their strengths and previous successes to overcome challenges. Such an approach to feedback fosters comprehensive learner development that leaves a lasting impact on their higher education experience and their transition to the workforce.

Ultimately, while the skills required to provide effective feedback demand practice, employing a coaching approach can significantly optimise the feedback process's cognitive and emotional aspects, transforming it into a rich opportunity for meaningful learning and growth.

Discussion Starters

- How might coaching help my students take on feedback I am already giving?
- How can I better acknowledge how hard it can be for students to receive feedback?
- How can I normalise for students the difficulty of receiving feedback?
- How is the negativity bias affecting the way I give feedback? How can I ensure I look for and share strengths in my feedback?
- How can I help students shift into a growth mindset regarding feedback?
- Where can I start adding more coaching to support giving feedback to my students?
- How can I share this with my colleagues?
- How can my students use these ideas for group work/peer feedback?

References

Boud, D., & Molloy, E. (2012). Rethinking models of feedback for learning: The challenge of design. *Assessment & Evaluation in Higher Education, 38*(6), 698–712. https://doi.org/10.1080/02602938.2012.691462

Crocker, J., & Luhtanen, R. (2003). Level of self-esteem and contingencies of self-worth: Unique effects on academic, social, and financial problems in college students. *Personality and Social Psychology Bulletin, 29*(6), 701–712. https://doi.org/10.1177/0146167203029006003

Dhawan, M. (2021, May 18). *A powerful ICF core competency: Embodies a coaching mindset.* International Coaching Federation. https://coachingfederation.org/blog/embodies-a-coaching-mindset

Dweck, C. (2006). *Mindset: The new psychology of success.* Random House.

Jackel, B., Pearce, J., Radloff, A., & Edwards, D. (2017). *Assessment and feedback in higher education: A review of literature for the higher education academy.* Higher Education Academy. https://research.acer.edu.au/higher_education/53

Jackson, P. Z., & McKergow, M. (2007). *The solutions focus: Making coaching and change simple* (2nd ed.). Nicholas Brealey Publishing.

Lieberman, M. D., Eisenberger, N. I., Crockett, M. J., Tom, S. M., Pfeifer, J. H., & Way, B. M. (2007). Putting feelings into words. *Psychological Science, 18*(5), 421–428. https://doi.org/10.1111/j.1467-9280.2007.01916.x

Linley, P. A., Nielsen, K. M., Wood, A. M., Gillett, R., & Biswas-Diener, R. (2010). Using signature strengths in pursuit of goals: Effects on goal progress, need satisfaction, and well-being, and implications for coaching psychologists. *International Coaching Psychology Review, 5*(1), 6–15. https://doi.org/10.53841/bpsicpr.2010.5.1.6

Lipnevich, A. A., & Panadero, E. (2021). A review of feedback models and theories: Descriptions, definitions, and conclusions. *Frontiers in Education, 6.* https://doi.org/10.3389/feduc.2021.720195

Orsmond, P., Maw, S. J., Park, J. R., Gomez, S., & Crook, A. C. (2011). Moving feedback forward: Theory to practice. *Assessment & Evaluation in Higher Education, 38*(2), 240–252. https://doi.org/10.1080/02602938.2011.625472

Paris, B. M. (2022). Instructors' perspectives of challenges and barriers to providing effective feedback. *Teaching and Learning Inquiry, 10.* https://doi.org/10.20343/teachlearninqu.10.3

Reynolds, M. (2020). *Coach the person, not the problem: A guide to use reflective inquiry.* Berrett-Koehler Publishers.

Rozin, P., & Royzman, E. B. (2001). Negativity bias, negativity dominance, and contagion. *Personality and Social Psychology Review, 5*(4), 296–320. https://doi.org/10.1207/s15327957pspr0504_2

Sadler, I., Reimann, N., & Sambell, K. (2022). Feedforward practices: A systematic review of the literature. *Assessment & Evaluation in Higher Education, 48*(3), 305–320. https://doi.org/10.1080/02602938.2022.2073434

Sargeant, J., Armson, H., Driessen, E., Holmboe, E., Könings, K., Lockyer, J., Lynn, L., Mann, K., Ross, K., Silver, I., Soklaridis, S., Warren, A., Zetkulic, M., Boudreau, M., & Shearer, C. (2016). Evidence-informed facilitated feedback: The R2C2 feedback model. *MedEdPORTAL.* https://doi.org/10.15766/mep_2374-8265.10387

Seko, Y., & Lau, P. (2021). Solution-focused approach in higher education: A scoping review. *Higher Education Research and Development, 41*(5), 1710–1726. https://doi.org/10.1080/07294360.2021.1920893

Tyng, C. M., Amin, H. U., Saad, M. N. M., & Malik, A. S. (2017). The influences of emotion on learning and memory. *Frontiers in Psychology, 8.* https://doi.org/10.3389/fpsyg.2017.01454

6 Coaching to Promote Retention

Supporting Academically At-Risk Students

Karina Dancza, May Sok Mui Lim and Kyrin Liong

Chapter Objectives

- To provide an understanding of the factors contributing to academic struggles among higher education students and identify students considered "at-risk" and in need of coaching support.
- To introduce the PROPER Coaching Framework as a practical tool for conducting coaching conversations with at-risk students.
- To address the importance of academic coaches' self-care and wellbeing in working with at-risk students in higher education.

Keywords

academic wellbeing
at-risk students
coaching framework
learning approaches
retention
self-efficacy

> The way a body looks, says nothing about its strength, its longevity, its endurance.
>
> Donna Ashworth

Introduction

Academic struggles among students can have various causes. They may be associated with multiple contextual factors, including financial pressures, housing concerns and family responsibilities. These external circumstances can significantly affect students' academic performance and individual factors like time management, self-regulation and study methods. This chapter discusses identifying "at-risk" students and guides when to initiate coaching conversations.

DOI: 10.4324/9781003332176-8

It includes examples of individual and group coaching approaches to help students overcome challenges and stay on track with their studies.

Additionally, the chapter explores the integration of learning analytics and coaching to support at-risk students. A practical guide, the PROPER Coaching Framework (Dancza et al., 2022a), is introduced to assist educators in conducting coaching conversations with students. Finally, the chapter addresses the wellbeing of academics who coach students and offers suggestions for maintaining self-care in the face of student complexities.

Introducing Jamie

Throughout this chapter, we will delve into various coaching approaches that can support students at risk of academic failure or withdrawal from higher education for various reasons. Drawing on our own experiences as university educators in Engineering (Kyrin) and Occupational Therapy (Karina and May), we will use the story of Jamie to illustrate some of the ideas presented.

Jamie is a first-year undergraduate engineering student with an impressive academic background, completing a three-year polytechnic course in offshore engineering with excellent grades. Before returning to academia, he served in the local military for two years. Being the first in his family to attend university, Jamie is enthusiastic about this new chapter. He envisions his degree financially supporting his parents and two younger siblings and boosting his self-esteem. However, he finds the first two weeks of the engineering course quite intense. For more details on Jamie's coaching journey and his challenges, please refer to Box 6.1, where he discusses his concerns with his classmate Sabrina.

Box 6.1   Jamie Sharing His Challenges with His Classmate Sabrina

Jamie: Oh my goodness, look at the things I'm supposed to remember from way back! I feel like my mind is still stuck in the jungle. But everyone else looks like they know what they're doing. I feel like I only know how to scroll through my social media feed.
    Hey Sabrina, is it just me? Cos I've just gotten back from two years in the Army or is this stuff really tough?

Sabrina: It's not you. I'm fresh from polytechnic and still I find it difficult. I've heard others saying the same thing too. Do you think maybe we should go speak to the professors?

Jamie: Hmmm, I don't know. I don't want to bother them. I feel like I can't quite get the concepts, but it's more than that. I don't have time to practise all these extra exercises when I go home because I need to help my parents and siblings with housework and earn money doing food deliveries in the evenings. I can't really afford fancy books, either. But how am I supposed to tell the professors that? It has nothing to do with lecture material.

Jamie's experience of feeling overwhelmed and uncertain when starting university is all too common, not just for students but anyone going through a significant life change. While some level of uncertainty is normal, it becomes a problem when it becomes too intense, making the student feel unable to cope, shutting down or even leading to dropping out of the program.

Research has identified various difficulties that first-year students face during the transition to university, including time management, overwhelming workload, subject difficulty, pressure from others' expectations, unpreparedness for university teaching style and increased responsibility for learning (Brooker et al., 2017; De Clercq et al., 2018; Kahu & Picton, 2020). While some students adapt well after the initial transition, others may try to brush their problems aside and hope that somehow it will work itself out, a likely ineffective strategy and one that can lead to failing courses and escalating the situation to a point where the university's policies decide if the student can continue or not.

As educators, we can make a difference through coaching conversations. However, asking for help can be challenging for students. Creating a safe and open conversation culture could encourage more students to seek help. By providing guidance, students can learn to (i) reflect on their emotions, rather than suppressing them (John & Gross, 2004), (ii) work through their emotions, rather than ignoring them (Attard, 2020), and if needed, (iii) take a break to heal instead of persisting through every challenging moment (Weir, 2019).

This chapter will explore coaching approaches for students who risk failing or withdrawing from higher education. We will focus on understanding these students beyond the classroom and, through coaching relationships, helping students take the next step toward a clearer self-vision of strong, resilient individuals. We will examine the type of at-risk students, how coaching can help, and explore coaching in group and individual settings.

Who Are the At-Risk Students?

According to Abrams and Jernigan (1984), "at-risk" students are commonly defined as more likely to perform poorly academically. At the university level, these students are often identified by a history of underperforming either in pre-university education (Polansky et al., 1993) or in their initial semesters (e.g. Abele et al., 2013; Young et al., 2015).

However, a history of poor academic performance is not the sole indicator of subsequent underperformance. Over the years, extensive research has identified various factors in personality traits, motivation, self-regulated learning strategies, learning approaches and psychosocial contextual influences that can influence academic performance among tertiary-level students (Richardson et al., 2012). Among these factors, students' psychosocial context and learning approach are particularly relevant to the concerning patterns observed among our first-year students.

Suppose we think about Jamie's background in completing his polytechnic diploma with good grades and a period of compulsory military training (standard practice for men in Singapore). He may face challenges transitioning to the academic environment as a first-generation university student. Factors such as being out of the routine of studying for two years, financial and personal pressures, and family responsibilities may contribute to increased stress levels, potentially affecting his wellbeing and academic progress. Despite his enthusiasm for starting university and previous academic achievements, these factors could hinder his success.

Student wellness (the psychosocial context) has received much attention recently. Factors like study-related stress (Pluut et al., 2015; Robotham, 2008) and school burnout (Salmela-Aro & Read, 2017; Schaufeli et al., 2002) are associated with poorer academic performance. Kaplan et al. (2005) conducted a longitudinal study and found that study-related stress during junior high school affected academic performance three years later.

The main message is that relying solely on past poor academic performance to identify at-risk students needs to be revised, as other factors can also predict future underperformance. Educators need to recognise the diverse factors that can put students at academic risk and hinder their successful completion of studies. In the following section, we will delve into practical approaches and the appropriate timing for engaging in coaching conversations with at-risk students.

Deciding When to Have a Coaching Conversation

A coaching approach goes beyond simply teaching concepts to struggling students; it can benefit all students by enhancing their learning strategies and approaches. However, the challenge lies in determining the timing of coaching conversations with at-risk students. Should it be initiated at the first signs of potential risk or when students face difficulties? Alternatively, could it be integrated as a routine practice to ensure all students benefit from coaching support?

Self-efficacy theory emphasises the impact of personal experiences on individuals' perception of their abilities (Bandura, 1977). Academic setbacks can significantly diminish students' confidence in their abilities, leading to lower self-efficacy, which in turn affects their performance negatively (Honicke & Broadbent, 2016; Pajares, 1996; Sitzmann & Yeo, 2013; Talsma et al., 2018; Zimmerman et al., 1992). Without support, at-risk students may spiral downward as poor performance reinforces their reduced self-efficacy. Understanding the link between self-efficacy and academic performance can guide the appropriate timing for coaching conversations.

Based on the authors' experience, early coaching conversations with students are more effective. Instead of waiting for students to reach a point of failure, engaging in coaching discussions with those who exhibit signs of struggle, such as late assignment submissions or disengagement during class activities, is more effective. Delaying intervention may lead to decreased self-efficacy and impact retention rates, making it essential to address concerns proactively. We share some examples in Box 6.2 illustrating that coaching conversations can benefit all students.

Box 6.2   Examples of When an Early Coaching Conversation Supported Students' Learning

1 I had a coaching conversation with a student who submitted an assignment two days late, which was a sign that she was not coping well after returning to study following many years in the workforce. The coaching conversation focused on time management and setting up an accountability partner, followed by a second coaching conversation to check progress. The student changed her study plan, stayed in the programme and successfully graduated with her class.
2 I was coaching a first-year student who felt burnt out. Through our conversations, I learned that the student had high expectations of herself and expected to excel in every subject. She gave up all leisure activities and sports to focus solely on her studies. Coaching conversations took place on managing her expectations and helping her gain a more holistic and meaningful university experience. She returned to playing sports and pursuing her interests, becoming more balanced and effective in studying.
3 The third example involved teaching in a team-based learning class with weekly small weightage quizzes. After coaching conversations with a handful of students who failed three quizzes, they identified new learning strategies that suited their learning styles. These students not only passed the course but also discovered better approaches to learning, which they applied to other courses.

The examples provided show no universally "perfect" time for all students to have initial coaching conversations. Instead, the ideal timing varies for each student, depending on their circumstances. Although coaching is often conducted individually, as educators, we frequently interact with students in group settings, so this may provide a natural starting point for coaching conversations.

Coaching At-Risk Students in a Group

Group coaching provides a supportive environment where students can act as accountability partners, working together towards achievable goals. It helps address issues like setting unrealistic expectations, struggling with accountability and difficulty moving past failures. In these conversations, students realise they are not alone and can offer each other valuable solutions and support.

In group supervision, educators may face situations where they oversee diverse groups of students working on projects. Each student brings unique strengths and needs, leading to challenges when some members feel their contributions are not fairly distributed. Additionally, some students may have social difficulties or a history of struggling with group work. Instead of singling out at-risk students for individual support, using coaching questions at the project's beginning fosters a healthy and inclusive group environment. This approach sets clear expectations and promotes accountability within the group. Box 6.3 provides some examples of coaching questions that can be used in this context.

Box 6.3   Coaching Questions to Set Group Expectations

1 What would you like to achieve at the end of this project? Apart from passing, what is your preferred future outcome?
2 Share one positive feedback or comment your friends gave you when working in groups.
3 If your previous group members were to offer you some well-intended advice, what do you think they would say?
4 How would you like the group to operate and function during the project?
5 What are some ways to maintain accountability among group members?
6 Have you experienced stressful group projects in the past? If so, what strategies or techniques have you used to manage the stress?
7 If, or when, issues arise in a group project relating to an individual's contribution, what is the best way to communicate this with you?
8 When reflecting on the project at the end, what would you like to feel most proud of?

Academic mentorship programmes in universities also offer valuable support to students, with professors, other university staff members or more senior students assigned as mentors to small groups. Some universities formalise such coaching and learning support through their student services. For instance, our university offers a programme called "Learning to Learn Better" for students facing study challenges. This programme involves an educator leading a small group of students in learning study skills, creating learning plans and understanding factors that impact learning. After group sessions, students receive individual coaching (see Chapter 12). These regular meetings allow mentors to provide tailored coaching, such as reflection on learning strategies after receiving results or stress management before exams. These conversations help students develop effective strategies for success without feeling singled out or labelled as "at-risk".

Another approach to supporting at-risk students involves data analytics. By identifying students with low Grade Point Averages or academic warnings, educators can offer group coaching sessions based on their past performance. Additionally, technology, such as analytics on the learning management system, can be used to monitor student engagement and progress in online learning environments. Educators can identify students needing extra support by tracking access to learning materials, sign-ins, and formative task completion. Group coaching allows students to share everyday struggles and develop strategies for better engagement with learning. While these indicators may not directly signal that a student is at risk, they allow educators to reach out and understand how the student is coping (Lim, 2021).

Coaching At-Risk Students Individually

Sometimes, we need to transition from group to individual coaching. The strengths-based perspective (Bannink, 2007) remains valuable when offering personalised support to students. This approach centres on identifying and leveraging their strengths to improve their situation. If something is not working, it encourages exploring alternative strategies. When dealing with challenging student situations, the strengths-based approach can effectively enhance the educator–student relationship and move them towards progress and improved coping (Dancza et al., 2022b).

Many coaching tools are available to guide a coaching conversation with students. One resource that one of the chapter's authors (Karina) developed for use in supervision is the **PROPER Coaching Framework** (Dancza et al., 2022a, p. 148). Each letter describes how a coach would move through a coaching conversation: Priority, Reality, Opportunity, Planning, Evaluate and Review (see Figure 6.1).

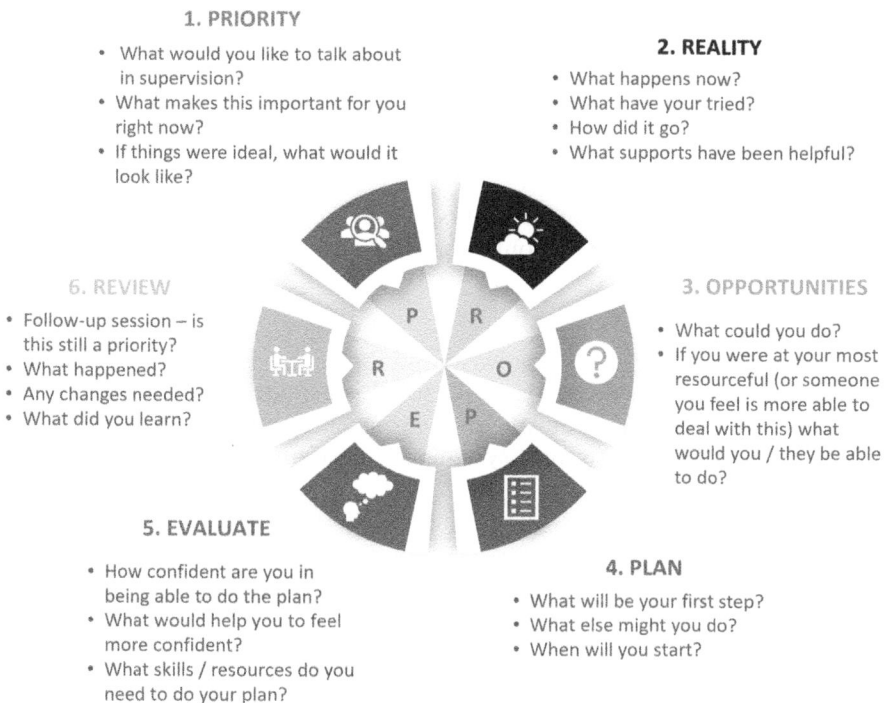

1. PRIORITY
- What would you like to talk about in supervision?
- What makes this important for you right now?
- If things were ideal, what would it look like?

2. REALITY
- What happens now?
- What have your tried?
- How did it go?
- What supports have been helpful?

6. REVIEW
- Follow-up session – is this still a priority?
- What happened?
- Any changes needed?
- What did you learn?

3. OPPORTUNITIES
- What could you do?
- If you were at your most resourceful (or someone you feel is more able to deal with this) what would you / they be able to do?

5. EVALUATE
- How confident are you in being able to do the plan?
- What would help you to feel more confident?
- What skills / resources do you need to do your plan?

4. PLAN
- What will be your first step?
- What else might you do?
- When will you start?

Figure 6.1 The PROPER Coaching Framework (Dancza et al., 2022a, p. 148)

Note: Used with permission of INFORMA UK LIMITED, Applying occupational therapy knowledge and skills to enhance supervision, p. 148, Figure 7.1 PROPER Coaching for Supervision Framework. From "Applying occupational therapy knowledge and skills to enhance supervision", by K. Dancza, S. Harvey, A. O'Dea, A. Volkert, & M. Penman, in K. Dancza, A. Volkert, & S. Tempest (Eds), *Supervision for occupational therapy: Practical guidance for supervisors and supervisees* (1st ed., p. 148), 2022, Routledge. Reproduced with permission of The Licensor through PLSclear.

As an integral component of our PROPER Coaching Framework (Dancza et al., 2022a), we have compiled a list of questions to help you during student conversations. These questions are designed to spark meaningful discussions and support students as they navigate their academic journey. Feel free to use and adapt them for more effective and empowering conversations with your students.

Priority

- What would you like to discuss today?
- What inspired you to choose this course of study?
- How do you define success in your academic journey?

Reality

- Can you identify some of your strengths contributing to your progress so far?
- What positive changes would you notice if you were coping better with your studies?
- On a scale of 1 to 10, with 1 representing very poor coping and 10 representing a high level of coping, where would you place yourself currently?
- What would that look like if you were to improve your coping by one point?

Opportunities

- Which learning strategies have been effective for you in the past, and are they still working?
- How can you leverage your strengths as a learner to make positive changes?
- Who are some people you could approach for support or learning opportunities?

Plan

- What immediate action can you take to initiate a positive change?
- What achievable things can you set for yourself to make progress?
- Are any resources or support systems available on or off campus to assist you with your studies?

Evaluate

- How confident do you feel about your plan, and what could increase your confidence?
- What specific support or assistance would you like from me to help you with your plan?

Review

- What progress or changes have you experienced since our last conversation?
- Is this still a priority for you?
- Are any adjustments needed to your current plan?

To illustrate how the PROPER Coaching Framework (Dancza et al., 2022a) might be used to structure a coaching conversation, we return to Jamie (Box 6.4). Jamie has been facing challenges with declining motivation and lower grades in his studies, and he is considering quitting to support his family financially after his mother's stroke. Professor Holly, concerned about Jamie's well-being, initiates a coaching conversation with him using the first five steps of the PROPER Coaching Framework.

Box 6.4 Using the Proper Coaching Framework in Conversation with Jamie

Prof Holly:	How are you, Jamie?
Jamie:	I have been better, professor. You know my grades aren't great at the moment.
Prof Holly:	Yes, that is why I wanted to chat with you. Are you OK to discuss this right now?
Jamie:	Hmm, yeah I guess
Prof Holly (Priority):	OK, so tell me what you think is the main challenge for you right now?
Jamie:	I don't really know … well my mum had a stroke and I have been caring for her when I can. I just can't seem to make any time to study. My mind just doesn't focus, and I feel overwhelmed.
Prof Holly:	That sounds tough, and I am sorry to hear about your mum.
Jamie:	Thanks. She is improving, but it has been hard on the whole family.
Prof Holly:	It is great to hear she is improving! Would you like to talk about your study routine to see if we can work out a plan together that might help you get back on track?
Jamie:	Yeah … that would be good. But I don't really know where to start.
Prof Holly (Reality):	Would you like to take me through what happens now when you try and study?
Jamie:	Well, I tend to start quite late, around 10 pm when the house is quiet. I then try to go through what we have done in class and recall what I am meant to do. I then feel overwhelmed and distract myself by flicking through my social media. Before I

	know it, it is past 2 am, and I decide to go to sleep.
Prof Holly (Opportunities):	OK, so what do you think you could do that would make a positive difference?
Jamie:	Hmmm … I could try and start earlier, I guess.
Prof Holly:	I will make a note of that. Is there anything else you could do?
Jamie:	The house is very busy, and I get distracted before people go to bed, so maybe I should try and stay back at university to study rather than try to do it at home?
Prof Holly:	I can add that idea to the list too. What about your friends, someone who you feel has a good studying routine, what do you think they would do in this situation?
Jamie:	Well, Sabrina is really efficient when studying. She always makes a note at the end of class as to what she needs to do next. I guess that means she has a plan of what to study so she can get straight to it. That might be worth a try? [Jamie and Holly continue to explore opportunities about what could change, with Holly asking targeted questions but not taking over and sharing her own suggestions.]
Prof Holly (Plan):	So we have generated a list of ideas. What do you want to try first?
Jamie:	I think I will try make a note at the end of class of what I need to do so I have a starting point for studying. Maybe I can also arrange with my brother to be with Mum on Tuesdays and Thursdays so I can stay back at university to study.
Prof Holly:	When do you think is realistic to start this?
Jamie:	I could make the list immediately in my next class … I might need a week or so to arrange with my brother to stay back at university.
Prof Holly (Evaluate):	Sounds like a plan. How confident are you to carry out your plan, on a scale of 1–10, where 1 is not at all confident and 10 is extremely confident?

Jamie:	I'd say about 7.
Prof Holly:	OK, what would make you an 8 or 9?
Jamie:	Hmm, I don't know how my brother might react as he has his own life too. Maybe if I had a backup plan, such as coming in a bit earlier to study when my lectures start after 10 am.
Prof Holly:	Good to have a plan B. Is there anything I could do to support you?
Jamie:	Would it be OK if I emailed you an update next week? I would like to see how I go, but it might be good to have a chat next month too?
Prof Holly:	Yes, happy to. I will wait for your email and please do let me know if you want to arrange another chat.
Jamie:	Thank you so much. I appreciate you checking in with me.

In this scenario, the professor took the initiative to approach Jamie, utilising the PROPER Coaching Framework (Dancza et al., 2022a) to structure a productive conversation. While Professor Holly could not directly address Jamie's home-related issues, guiding him to create an academic improvement plan was significant.

As educators, it is crucial to acknowledge our limitations and recognise when students may require support from trained professionals like counsellors or psychologists who possess expertise in specific areas. Coaching a student to take action in seeking professional help could be an important goal. Additionally, taking care of our wellbeing and seeking support when necessary is important. We will discuss this further in the next section.

Support for Educators Who Coach

Educators often prioritise the safety and progress of their students above all else, despite being aware of the potential negative impact on their own wellbeing (McGuffog et al., 2021). This emotional involvement in supporting and guiding students can become overwhelming. To address this, educators and coaches must build a supportive community around themselves to stay grounded (Kaplan, 2022). Box 6.5 presents a conversation between Professor Holly and her colleague, shedding light on how these emotions may manifest in practice.

Box 6.5   Holly's (Jamie's Professor) Conversation with Her Colleague on Jamie's Progress

Colleague: Hey Holly, how are you doing with your student Jamie, who's going through a rough patch?

Holly: Jamie's doing better; he seems to be working through things quite well.

Colleague: OK, that's good news. How are you doing?

Holly: I've been feeling a little tired – nothing to worry about. I'm glad Jamie is doing well. Maybe this class has taken quite a lot of my energy ....

Box 6.5 illustrates the importance of simple check-ins among colleagues, as it offers valuable support to educators like Holly, who may be dealing with struggling students. These interactions create a healthy coaching community where experiences can be shared and mutual support is provided.

Forming a community of colleagues also brings benefits in understanding challenging situations. For example, when coaching students like Jamie, there is a risk of not achieving the desired progress, leading to feelings of disappointment and failure. However, colleagues can provide an external and unbiased perspective, clarifying thoughts and offering fresh insights (Brookefield, 2006). While they may not always offer new solutions, their input serves as a sounding board to identify blind spots and view the situation more positively.

Creating a community of colleagues and friends offers several advantages in supporting educators as they guide at-risk students. Though each situation is unique, sharing the anxieties and insecurities that come with being a coach in higher education can be helpful (Eveleigh et al., 2022). This shared perspective can bring relief and clarity, fostering a space where solutions are collectively sought for common challenges.

Coaching can also be a powerful tool for supporting each other as educators within a professional community. Educators can engage in meaningful conversations that promote self-reflection, active listening, and empathetic understanding by adopting a coaching approach. Through these interactions, educators can share experiences, challenges, and successes, creating a supportive and collaborative environment. Coaching allows educators to explore their strengths and areas for growth, fostering a culture of continuous learning and improvement. Through coaching, educators can build trust, develop strong connections, and form a community of support, ensuring that they are better equipped to meet the diverse needs of their students and maintain their own wellbeing in the demanding field of education. By looking out for one another, educators can recognise when someone needs a break to recharge, emphasising the importance of prioritising their own wellbeing (McGuffog et al., 2021). Practicing self-care enables educators to show up fully for their students, offering the necessary support they deserve. It's important to know that self-care is not a selfish act but good stewardship for us to be available for those we care about.

Conclusion

This chapter delved into the multifaceted nature of academic struggles among students, which could have various causes. The chapter offered practical advice on effectively engaging students in coaching discussions, highlighting both individual and group coaching approaches that could be instrumental in helping students overcome obstacles and maintain academic progress. A comprehensive coaching framework, known as the PROPER Coaching Framework (Dancza et al., 2022a), was introduced to provide educators with a structured approach to conducting coaching conversations and fostering student success. Recognising the potential challenges faced by educators in their role as coaches, the chapter also addressed the importance of self-care and wellbeing. It offered suggestions and strategies to help educators maintain their own emotional and mental wellbeing while navigating the complexities of supporting at-risk students.

Discussion Starters

Below are some conversation starters and coaching questions that can assist educators in reflecting on their practice, identifying areas for growth and development, and improving their support for all students, including those who may be considered 'at-risk'.

- What strategies have you tried so far when coaching at-risk students?
- Have these strategies been effective? If not, what can be done differently?
- Who else can you consult or seek advice from to improve your coaching with at-risk students?
- What specific feedback or guidance would you like to receive to enhance your coaching abilities?
- How would you know when it is time to ask for help or seek feedback when coaching at-risk students?
- How confident are you in implementing new strategies or changing your current coaching approach?
- What additional resources or training might you need to feel more confident in coaching at-risk students effectively?

References

Abele, C., Penprase, B., & Ternes, R. (2013). A closer look at academic probation and attrition: What courses are predictive of nursing student success? *Nurse Education Today*, *33*(3), 258–261. https://doi.org/10.1016/J.NEDT.2011.11.017

Abrams, H. G., & Jernigan, L. P. (1984). Academic support services and the success of high-risk college students. *American Educational Research Journal*, *21*(2), 261–274. https://doi.org/10.3102/00028312021002261

Attard, A. (2020, November 4). *Repressing emotions: 10 ways to reduce emotional avoidance*. PositivePsychology.com. https://positivepsychology.com/repress-emotions/

Bandura, A. (1977). Self-efficacy: Toward a unifying theory of behavioral change. *Advances in Behaviour Research and Therapy*, *1*(4), 139–161. https://doi.org/10.1016/0146-6402(78)90002-4

Bannink, F. P. (2007). Solution-focused brief therapy. *Journal of Contemporary Psychotherapy, 37*(2), 87–94. https://doi.org/10.1007/s10879-006-9040-y

Brookefield, S.D. (2006). *The skillful teacher: On technique, trust and responsiveness in the classroom* (2nd ed.). Jossey-Bass.

Brooker, A., Brooker, S., & Lawrence, J. (2017). First year students' perceptions of their difficulties. *Student Success, 8*(1), 49–62. https://doi.org/10.5204/ssj.v8i1.352

Dancza, K., Harvey, S., O'Dea, A., Volkert, A., Penman, M., & Kennedy-Behr, A. (2022a). Applying occupational therapy knowledge and skills to enhance supervision. In K. Dancza, A. Volkert, & S. Tempest (Eds), *Supervision for occupational therapy: Practical guidance for supervisors and supervisees* (pp. 143–168): Routledge. https://doi.org/10.4324/9781003092544-7

Dancza, K., Tempest, S., Baird, J. M., Volkert, A., Sajid, M., & Kramer-Roy, D. (2022b). Concepts that help us do supervision well. In K. Dancza, A. Volkert, & S. Tempest (Eds), *Supervision for occupational therapy: Practical guidance for supervisors and supervisees* (pp. 25–47). Routledge. https://doi.org/10.4324/9781003092544-2

De Clercq, M., Roland, N., Brunelle, M., Galand, B., & Frenay, M. (2018). The delicate balance to adjustment: A qualitative approach of student's transition to the first year at university. *Psychologica Belgica, 58*(1), 67–90. https://doi.org/10.5334/pb.409

Eveleigh, A., Cook, A., Naples, L. H., & Cipriano, C. (2022). How did educators of students with learning differences use social–emotional learning to support their students and themselves early in the covid-19 pandemic? *Children & Schools, 44*(1), 27–38. https://doi.org/10.1093/cs/cdab030

Honicke, T., & Broadbent, J. (2016). The influence of academic self-efficacy on academic performance: A systematic review. *Educational Research Review, 17*, 63–84. https://doi.org/10.1016/J.EDUREV.2015.11.002

John, O. P., & Gross, J. J. (2004). Healthy and unhealthy emotion regulation: Personality processes, individual differences, and life span development. *Journal of Personality, 72*(6), 1301–1334. https://doi.org/10.1111/j.1467-6494.2004.00298.x

Kahu, E. R., & Picton, C. (2020). Using photo elicitation to understand first-year student experiences: Student metaphors of life, university and learning. *Active Learning in Higher Education, 23*(1), 35–47. https://doi.org/10.1177/1469787420908384

Kaplan, D. S., Liu, R. X., & Kaplan, H. B. (2005). School related stress in early adolescence and academic performance three years later: The conditional influence of self expectations. *Social Psychology of Education, 8*(1), 3–17. https://doi.org/10.1007/s11218-004-3129-5

Kaplan, H. (2022). The unique effects of supporting beginning teachers' psychological needs through learning communities and a teacher-mentor's support: A longitudinal study based on self-determination theory. *Frontiers in Psychology, 13*. https://doi.org/10.3389/fpsyg.2022.859364

Lim, S. M. (2021, February 1). *Use technology to catch students before they fall*. Times Higher Education. www.timeshighereducation.com/campus/use-technology-catch-students-they-fall

McGuffog, R., Fitzgeraldson, E., Lyford, B., Triandafilidis, Z., Fitzpatrick, S., & Hazel, G. (2021). Australian family day care educators' experiences of supporting children's mental health, and their own mental health and wellbeing. *Australasian Journal of Early Childhood, 47*(2), 107–120. https://doi.org/10.1177/18369391211063663

Pajares, F. (1996). Self-efficacy beliefs in academic settings. *Review of Educational Research, 66*(4), 543–578. https://doi.org/10.3102/00346543066004543

Pluut, H., Curşeu, P. L., & Ilies, R. (2015). Social and study related stressors and resources among university entrants: Effects on well-being and academic performance. *Learning and Individual Differences, 37*, 262–268. https://doi.org/10.1016/J.LINDIF.2014.11.018

Polansky, J., Horan, J. J., & Hanish, C. (1993). Experimental construct validity of the outcomes of study skills training and career counseling as treatments for the retention of at-risk students. *Journal of Counseling & Development, 71*(5), 488–492. https://doi.org/10.1002/j.1556-6676.1993.tb02230.x

Richardson, M., Abraham, C., & Bond, R. (2012). Psychological correlates of university students' academic performance: A systematic review and meta-analysis. *Psychological Bulletin, 138*(2), 353–387. https://doi.org/10.1037/a0026838

Robotham, D. (2008). Stress among higher education students: Towards a research agenda. *Higher Educatin, 56*(6), 735–746. https://doi.org/10.1007/s10734-008-9137-1

Salmela-Aro, K., & Read, S. (2017). Study engagement and burnout profiles among Finnish higher education students. *Burnout Research, 7*, 21–28. https://doi.org/10.1016/J.BURN.2017.11.001

Schaufeli, W. B., Martínez, I. M., Pinto, A. M., Salanova, M., & Bakker, A. B. (2002). Burnout and engagement in university students: A cross-national study. *Journal of Cross-Cultural Psychology, 33*(5), 464–481. https://doi.org/10.1177/0022022102033005003

Sitzmann, T., & Yeo, G. (2013). A meta-analytic investigation of the within-person self-efficacy domain: Is self-efficacy a product of past performance or a driver of future performance? *Personnel Psychology, 66*(3), 531–568. https://doi.org/10.1111/peps.12035

Talsma, K., Schüz, B., Schwarzer, R., & Norris, K. (2018). I believe, therefore I achieve (and vice versa): A meta-analytic cross-lagged panel analysis of self-efficacy and academic performance. *Learning and Individual Differences, 61*, 136–150. https://doi.org/10.1016/J.LINDIF.2017.11.015

Weir, K. (2019, January). Give me a break. *Monitor on Psychology, 50*(1), 40–41.

Young, T. L., Turnage-Butterbaugh, I., Degges-White, S., & Mossing, S. (2015). Wellness among undergraduate students on academic probation: Implications for college counselors. *Journal of College Counseling, 18*(3), 222–232. https://doi.org/10.1002/jocc.12016

Zimmerman, B. J., Bandura, A., & Martinez-Pons, M. (1992). Self-motivation for academic attainment: The role of self-efficacy beliefs and personal goal setting. *American Educational Research Journal, 29*(3), 663–676. https://doi.org/10.3102/00028312029003663

7 Using a Coaching Approach for Group Work

Holly Andrews

Chapter Objectives

- To identify why and how coaching can support effective group work in higher education.
- To explore some group dynamics that may impact how groups of students work together.
- To highlight how a solution-focused approach can be used to coach groups.
- To discuss the coachable moments that can occur in the lifespan of student groups.

Keywords

group coaching
group dynamics
group work
mirroring
psychological safety
strengths
stretching

Introduction

Humans are fundamentally social creatures; we live our lives in groups, including family, friendship, and work groups. These groups have the potential to be both extremely rewarding and to lead to negative emotions such as rejection, anxiety and fear (Forsyth, 2018). At university, students naturally form new groups and are often placed in artificial groups for group work. This chapter will focus on how coaching can facilitate group work at university.

At the outset, we need to consider the definition of a group and how this differs from a team. All teams are groups, but not all groups are teams. Groups

DOI: 10.4324/9781003332176-9

can consist of individuals who come together for some purpose (e.g. people at a concert). However, they do not necessarily share a common goal (e.g. some people may want to listen to music, some dance, others enjoy time with friends). In contrast, a team has a shared goal, and the achievement of that goal depends upon the individual actions of team members (e.g. a football team winning a match is dependent on the contributions of the whole team) (Thornton, 2016). In some ways, our groups of students operate as a team in that they have a shared project requiring collaboration. However, the team will have a limited lifespan that ends when the project is completed and they no longer share common goals. This gives our student groups a unique blend of team and group characteristics, as discussed later in the chapter. Throughout the chapter, the terms group and team will be used interchangeably to refer to groups of students working towards a common goal for a limited time.

Group Work in Higher Education (HE)

Many universities utilise group work as part of their pedagogy and assessment strategy (Volet & Mansfield, 2006). Working well with others is one of the most frequently cited skills requested by graduate employers (Osmani et al., 2019). Universities, therefore, attempt to develop students' teamwork skills by providing opportunities for students to work together in groups on projects, assuming that this will enhance students' skills.

Problems in Developing Teamworking Skills

There are three main issues with this approach. First, teamwork is not an easy skill to master, and many students arrive at university without developing adequate teamwork skills. By setting group tasks, we ask students to do something they must be equipped for. As any tutor who has supervised group work will attest, problems inevitably arise in many groups. Those groups then need to capitalise on the potential of the individual group members and perform below their capabilities. Second, students are not supported to develop teamwork when engaging in group projects at university, so the project's development potential is limited. The development of skills is often expected to occur through experience. According to Kolb's reflective learning cycle (Kolb, 2015), experiencing something is just one part of the learning process; one also needs to be able to reflect on that experience, draw meaning from it and plan new ways to act in the future in order to learn and develop. Third, where issues occur, tutors often step in to help the students to resolve the issues. This further limits the potential for students to learn and develop valuable teamwork skills. A student whose tutor has solved a group issue for them will not have developed the skills to solve a problem that occurs the next time they are working in a group.

A coaching approach to facilitating group work can help educators support students in developing their teamwork skills, resulting in better performance, more significant development of transferable skills and more satisfaction with group work. This chapter will examine some group dynamics that may be at play within group work at university and how these can impact effective teamwork. We will then look at how coaching can be used at various points in group work to help students understand themselves and others within their group and use this knowledge to improve their teamwork now and in the future.

Group Dynamics in Higher Education

In any group setting, many group dynamics are at play stemming from our innate needs as humans, the unique qualities and experiences of the individuals involved and the context in which the group operates. These dynamics have the potential to accelerate or hinder learning and development. Thornton (2016) identifies nine group processes. We explore three of these that most frequently occur when students are required to work together in HE. We also examine the concept of psychological safety and how it impacts student groups.

The Group Matrix

The group matrix refers to both the dynamic matrix and the foundation matrix. The dynamic matrix is the group's shared experiences that build up and change over time, leading to the group having an ever-evolving conscious and unconscious sense of this particular group. It might include what is acceptable to say and do in the group and what the group sees as "good". The foundation matrix includes both our innate drives as human beings and our cultural heritage. The foundation matrix may be evident in groups that include students from different cultural backgrounds where there may not necessarily be similar shared assumptions. For example, students may have different cultural approaches to challenge and critique.

When coaching a student group, the coach must know the dynamic matrix building up within the group and the foundation matrix within each individual. Considering what things mean for the group and the individual is therefore essential. Helping students communicate their values and assumptions verbally and what they are assuming about the group can help them avoid misunderstandings.

Mirroring

The brain is designed to help us learn from and identify with other humans. We know from neuroscience that mirror neurons are fired in both instances when we act and when we watch someone else act. For example, if you watch someone eating a delicious chocolate bar, do you salivate? There can be positive aspects of mirroring in a group, such as making us feel seen and understood, connecting us via shared experiences and understandings – *That is just like me!* – and helping us to see ourselves more clearly through the eyes of others.

Mirroring can also be detrimental. Projection can occur when we see aspects of ourselves in another group member that we do not like. Projecting these onto another person helps to distance us from aspects of ourselves that we would rather not have. For example, I might dislike how disorganised I am, and instead of acknowledging this trait in myself, I label another group member as disorganised. Transference occurs when we bring the dynamics from a previous relationship into a current one. For example, a student may have had an extremely competitive relationship with a sibling and is now highly competitive with a group member. Both projection and transference are often unconscious.

When coaching student groups, it is inappropriate to delve into past relationships or stray towards the boundary of therapy and coaching. Negative mirroring can be minimised by facilitating good communication in a group so unconscious processes can be identified by the group and dealt with. For example, the student who projects their procrastination habit onto a fellow group member may receive feedback from the rest of the group that helps them recognise this trait in *themselves*. The coach can then support the student in planning to deal with this.

Location and Scapegoating

Everything in a group, even if it appears to be focused on one individual, is a product of all the group members. For example, a group member who repeatedly misses deadlines may be labelled a problem. The problem may be multi-faceted, including the tardy individual's working habits, how realistic the group's deadlines are and what response has been received by people who speak up about any difficulties they are having. Particularly in groups experiencing challenges, it can be convenient to ascribe the issue to one or two individuals. A coach can help the group explore how everyone in the group is contributing to the issue and collectively work towards solving the problem.

Psychological Safety

Beyond group dynamics, psychological safety is another concept that is key to success in groups. Psychological safety refers to the extent to which individuals feel safe to take interpersonal risks, such as admitting when they do not know something, asking for help, challenging the group consensus, or requesting feedback (Edmondson, 1999). Psychological safety enables people to learn more in groups, as taking on challenging goals that allow for development is risky, and individuals will only engage in this if they feel that they will not suffer adverse consequences for failure or mistakes made.

A coach can help to facilitate psychological safety in a group. Initial contracting can make explicit things like what group members should do if they need clarification on something, how the group will respond to mistakes made and how feedback can be productively delivered to individuals in the group. Such agreements can lay the foundations for psychological safety. The coach can then check how the team upholds these agreements as the project progresses.

Now that we have examined the issues with group work in HE, we examine how a solution-focused approach to coaching can help student groups work more effectively and develop greater teamwork skills.

Solution-Focused Group Coaching in Higher Education

A solution-focused approach to coaching groups has many advantages in a HE context.

- Groups usually have a set task to complete together, so focusing on goals is appropriate.
- Often students need to learn about each other, so they may be reluctant to focus on discussing their weaknesses or what they perceive as the weaknesses of others in the group.
- As group work is usually time-limited in HE, moving quickly towards how to address a problem is advantageous.
- Focusing on moving towards a solution and avoiding problems avoid a blame culture in the group (O'Connell & Palmer, 2018).
- The group will learn valuable solution-focused skills that will improve their future teamwork.

Many good texts on group and team differentiate between the two types of coaching and make differing suggestions regarding how the coach should approach the assignment. The essence of the difference is that in group coaching, the group members do not have shared goals, are not a group outside of the coaching and do not have a shared history or future together. The opposite is true for team coaching. Student project groups in HE present as a unique hybrid of the two. The students will typically have a shared goal (e.g. completing a project or assignment set by the tutor) and will, therefore, be a team in this respect. However, groups are often put together to complete a task. Therefore, they need a team's shared history or future as defined in the coaching literature. Because of this, the educator needs to blend some of the approaches used with groups and teams when coaching groups of students.

The following sections cover the significant coachable moments in the life of student groups and outline how solution-focused group coaching can be applied in those moments.

Coaching Opportunities with Groups in Higher Education

This section covers four critical points in a group's life that offer coaching opportunities to make a significant impact; when groups first form, when groups experience problems, when groups are successful and when groups end.

When the Group First Forms

Many student groups take time to begin working together effectively. The tutor can use coaching to help the group navigate the tricky stages of group development of forming, norming and storming, where people are figuring out how the group will work together (Tuckman, 1965). Coaching sessions early in the life of groups can be used to facilitate the following situations:

- When students are getting to know one another: Some students are only willing to talk about themselves if instructed. The coach can provide a safe space for students to speak a little about themselves if they do not know the other group members. In a solution-focused approach, this should also include identifying strengths and resources. Some of the ways the coach can facilitate this are discussed below.
- During discussions on how the group will work together: When people need to gain experience working in teams, they often launch straight into the task without first considering how the group can best work together. The coach can ensure this discussion happens, often saving many problems further down the line.
- When resolving early frictions between group members. Different working styles, experience levels, cultures and personalities can make working together more challenging. A solution-focused approach can help students shift focus away from the difficulties they find in working together towards the strengths they can appreciate in others and the steps they can take towards working more effectively together.

Guidance for the First Coaching Session

O'Connell et al. (2012) outline several approaches and tools that can be used when coaching groups and teams. Based on their work, the table below outlines a suggested structure for a first coaching session that blends some of these into a structure that can work when coaching student groups. A workable structure/format to follow as suggested in Table 7.1 would be:

1 Contracting
2 Goal setting
3 Strength analysis
4 Strategy
5 Wrap-up

Table 7.1 First Coaching Session Structure

Stage	Activities
Contracting	As with any coaching assignment, contracting at the outset is essential. The dual role of tutor and coach can make it difficult for students to embrace the lack of direction provided in coaching (Jones & Andrews, 2019); therefore, making it clear that you will not be solving their problems for them will be necessary from the outset. You should explain what a solution-focused approach to coaching a group is (see Chapter 2) and how you will facilitate this approach. Work with the group to identify some ground rules of how they want to work together, both in the coaching sessions and outside. This can help students move towards the "norming" phase of group development (Tuckman, 1965).
Goal setting	While students will typically have a set assignment or project to work on as a group, there will usually still be some decisions they need to make about what they want to achieve. If there is a choice of topic, for example, what do they want to focus on? If the work is graded, what grade are they aiming for? This stage can also include the students considering how they want to work together as a team. One exercise that can help with this is profiling a solution-focused team. Now that the students have been introduced to the idea of being solution-focused, they can discuss what a "good" solution-focused team would look like. What would they notice about the team? What do the team members say and do? What values do they hold? How do they work with one another? What does it feel like to be a member of this team?
Strength analysis	Many of the exercises that are traditional in team solution-focused coaching, such as identifying past successes as a team, are not applicable at the start of a student group, as they have no shared history to work from. Here the coach needs to work with the group to help them identify their individual strengths and how they might be used in the group. Reviewing past group projects, they have independently been a part of the role they played, and their main contributions can help here. Using psychometrics (e.g. assessment tool for identifying strengths) can also facilitate this discussion.
Strategy	Solution-focused team coaching is all about moving the team forward in the pursuit of their goals. One exercise that might be useful with a student group is a version of de Shazer's (1988) miracle question. The coach can ask the students to imagine the project is complete and it has been a success. How would they know it had been successful? What would the team have done to achieve that success? How would they have communicated and interacted with each other? What behaviours would be seen in the group? The answers to these questions can help the group to identify how they need to tackle their project.
Wrap-up	Conclude the session with the students committing to the next steps they are going to take to move them towards their goals. When coaching students, you may need to be more directive than a coach normally would be, instructing the students to make a note of the actions they are agreeing to and when they need to complete them. The coach should also make a note of these. The students should also agree at this stage how they are going to support one another to achieve their individual actions.

Depending on the time allowed, the coach may not get to step 4 in the first coaching session with a group. This is fine; stage four is usually the focus for subsequent sessions.

Coaching questions for the first session:

- What do you want to achieve as a group?
- How will you work together effectively? What ground rules does the group need to have?
- What individual strengths do you bring to the group?
- What has made your past group work a success?

Once groups are established, they can offer different coaching opportunities, whether the group is experiencing problems or success.

When the Group Is Experiencing Problems

When groups have hit a block in their project, a coaching session can help students navigate through their options and test any assumptions they are making that may be blocking their progress. While hearing the problem is important, solution-focused coaching aims to move towards solutions rather than dwelling on the issues. Some specific coaching tools can be useful in this scenario:

1 Small steps. Present the group with two sheets of flip chart paper. Ask the group to write the problems they are experiencing on one sheet and the small steps they could take towards resolving the problems on the other. Then ask one person in the team to rip up the problem sheet. The group can then move away from the problem to discuss the possible steps they could take (O'Connell et al., 2012).
2 Four boxes. Use four pieces of flip chart paper and ask the group to work their way through the following on each piece; what is the issue; what is the preferred outcome; what resources do they have as a group; and what are the next steps they could take towards tackling the problem? (Korman, n.d., cited in O'Connell et al., 2012).

The case study in Box 7.1 illustrates one group where solution-focused coaching was used to help them overcome a major obstacle in their project.

Box 7.1   Charity Project Case Study

I ran a business module where students were tasked with designing and executing a fundraising project on behalf of a local charity. Within their groups, students had to assume a specific business role (e.g. marketing manager, finance manager) and adopt the responsibilities associated with that role for the project. The group work was assessed. Each student had to produce an individual piece of written work related to their role and the group was required to deliver a group presentation on the project. Students were able to choose who they worked with after five weeks of the course.

A group of four students were working on a balloon race to raise money for a local children's charity. The group were working well together. They had researched how to make a successful balloon race had gained approval for the project from the charity and had secured the backing of a high-profile local sports team, who would allow them to sell tickets at an upcoming match and launch the balloons at half-time. They launched their marketing plan, which included social media posts using the hashtag #balloonrace. What followed was completely unexpected. The group's posts were commented upon by individuals concerned about animal welfare. The University Vice Chancellor was also contacted directly by individuals to express their concern that the university was supporting a balloon race event. The decision was taken to rescind approval for the balloon race and the group were faced with a very short period in which to come up with a new project.

As their coach, I started the session by allowing them to talk about the problem they were experiencing and ensuring that they felt heard. Once they had been able to air their issues, I moved us to discuss what they wanted to achieve by the end of the coaching session. They wanted to have a new idea that they could action by the project deadline. I sensed that they felt deflated as a group, having put a lot of effort into the original balloon race, so it seemed important to me that we started with a focus on their strengths and resources. I asked them to identify the strengths other team members had shown when coming up with the original project (I noticed that students found it easier to identify strengths in others than in themselves). This led to a discussion of strengths they have shown in other situations when things had become difficult. This led us to write a list of all the strengths they had as a group that they could deploy in solving this problem. I was also careful to affirm their hard work so far and what they had achieved. The energy in the group shifted, and they were more confident that they could overcome this problem and find a new idea. Now they were in a position to brainstorm the steps that they could take towards solving the problem. As a next step, the group agreed that they would each spend one hour researching possible ideas and then meet to discuss these the following day.

The group decided on a virtual balloon race, which was a great success and made them one of the most successful groups ever on the module in terms of money raised.

There are some key learning points for the educator from this case study:

1 You cannot ignore problems in a solution-focused approach; groups must be heard.
2 Pay attention to the energy in a group. When groups are experiencing problems, you may need to spend some time building up their confidence.
3 Move towards small but positive actions, especially when a problem seems large. Taking small steps will help to build self-efficacy in the group.

Coaching questions for when the group is experiencing problems:

- When have you solved difficult problems in the past? What did you do?
- What small step could you take towards a solution to this problem?
- How could you use the strengths in this group to move you forward?

When Things Are Going Well for the Group

When groups are progressing well, giving them less time and attention can be tempting, leaving them to "get on with it". However, ensuring that students recognise what is going well for them and, more importantly, why can ensure that they remain motivated. It can also help if they run into a problem, as they can more readily access knowledge of what they were doing when they were successful and consider how they can apply this to solving the problem. Some activities you might consider using with successful groups include:

- Scaling. Place ten sheets of paper on the floor with the numbers 1–10. Ask each group member to stand by the number they think represents how well things are going at the moment, with 1 being the worst they can be and 10 being the best they can be. Ask each group member to explain their decision, which can help to uncover differing perspectives. Assuming that not everyone selected 10, the group can then discuss how to move one point up the scale (O'Connell et al., 2012).
- Stretching. Sometimes things are going well because the group has not selected a goal that challenges its members. If the current goal appears to be in hand, the coach can challenge the group to identify ways in which they could do just a little bit more and consequently achieve a little bit more in the project (O'Connell et al., 2012).

Coaching questions for when things are going well:

- What are you doing that is contributing to the group's success?
- How could you stretch yourself to achieve more?

At the End of the Group Project

Once a group project has finished, student groups often disband quickly, without the opportunity to reflect on the experience and consolidate the learning that has taken place. The coach can use a final coaching session as suggested in Table 7.2

Table 7.2 Final Coaching Session Structure

Stage	Activity
Review	The coach can allow some space for the students to review what has happened in the group. What have been the highs and the lows? What are they most proud of? How successful have they been in achieving their goals?
Appreciate	Asking students to share what they appreciated in their teammates keeps the discussion focused on positives rather than problems and avoids a blame culture.
Reflect	Giving students some time individually to reflect on what they have learnt from the experience.
Plan	The group can share what they will do the next time they are involved in a group project. The coach needs to use their skills to keep this focused on positive changes each group member can make.

to encourage this kind of learning to happen. Endings can also be challenging in themselves, as there are often both positive and negative feelings associated with the ending of a group. In this context, students may be worried about not having the support of the group in other work, or they may be happy to be moving onto something new. A coach can help to facilitate the expression of both positive and negative feelings. This can also be supported by the design of a module that requires some kind of reflective writing on the group work experience as part of the assessment.

The following questions can be use for the final coaching session:

• What have you learnt from your experiences in this group?
• What will you do in group work in the future?

Practicalities of Group Coaching

Coaching groups can be challenging, and it is very important to attend to the practical details to ensure the coaching goes as smoothly as possible. Some things to consider are listed below:

• Start and finish on time.
  Waiting for people to turn up or allowing the group to run over can cause resentment and frustration in a group, so be clear about your expectations regarding attendance and time keeping.
• Minimise distractions.
  The group need to be able to work together uninterrupted, so ask that mobile phones and other devices be switched off, so the group can focus on the coaching.
• Choose a quiet and comfortable space.

This can be a challenge in higher education, where room allocation is often not down to the academic, so explain your needs to the appropriate department as much as possible. A consistent place is also important so the group can finish their work before settling into a new environment each session. Finally, avoid using your office or a classroom, as these place you in a position of power and authority rather than a coaching role (Jones & Andrews, 2019).

Conclusion

It is generally accepted that teamwork is a valuable skill for students and is required in the job market. While university courses frequently include group work as part of the student experience, it is often not designed to ensure that students gain the maximum amount of learning and develop their teamwork skills. Teamworking is difficult, and there can be many unconscious processes at play that students are not equipped to manage. Taking a solution-focused approach to coaching student groups can provide the time and space for students to reflect on their experiences in their group, identify how they can best work together and solve any problems they may be experiencing. You can also facilitate students identifying how they can approach group work in the future to be better team members.

Coaching Questions

- What do you want to achieve as a group?
- How will you work together effectively? What ground rules does the group need to have?
- What individual strengths do you bring to the group?
- What has made your past group work a success?
- When have you solved difficult problems in the past? What did you do?
- What small step could you take towards a solution to this problem?
- How could you use the strengths in this group to move you forward?
- What are you doing that is contributing to the group's success?
- How could you stretch yourself to achieve more?
- What have you learnt from your experiences in this group?
- What will you do in group work in the future?

Summary

- Teamworking is an essential skill for students to develop, but more than providing opportunities for students to work in groups is needed for skill development.
- Group dynamics, including the group matrix, mirroring location and scapegoating, can negatively impact the ability of student groups to work together effectively and be a barrier to learning within a group environment. Psychological safety is also required for learning in groups to be maximised.

- A solution-focused approach to group coaching can help students to focus on their goals, recognise and use their strengths appropriately, and avoid excessive focus on problems.
- The start of a group project, when the group encounters difficulties, when the group is successful and at the end of a group project are all coachable moments when a solution-focused approach can be deployed.
- The group coach needs to allow the students to feel heard and then move towards reinforcing their self-efficacy by focusing on strengths and achievements and how they will move forward.
- Practical issues are also critical in group coaching, so timekeeping and location are essential.

Discussion Starters

- What issues have you encountered with student group work?
- How have you approached supporting student group work previously?
- How confidently can you notice group dynamics at play and support groups to navigate these? How could you become more confident?
- What coaching programme could you set up to support your student's group work?

References

de Shazer, S. (1988). *Clues: Investigating solutions in brief therapy*. W. W. Norton.

Edmondson, A. (1999). Psychological safety and learning behavior in work teams. *Administrative Science Quarterly*, *44*(2), 350–383. https://doi.org/10.2307/2666999

Forsyth, D. R. (2018). *Group dynamics* (7th ed.). Cengage Learning.

Jones, R. J., & Andrews, H. (2019). Understanding the rise of faculty–student coaching: An academic capitalism perspective. *Academy of Management Learning & Education*, *18*(4), 606–625. https://doi.org/10.5465/amle.2017.0200

Kolb, D. A. (2015). *Experiential learning: Experience as the source of learning and development* (2nd ed.). Pearson Education.

O'Connell, B., & Palmer, S. (2018). Solution-focused coaching. In S. Palmer & A. Whybrow (Eds), *Handbook of coaching psychology* (pp. 270–281). Routledge. https://doi.org/10.4324/9781315758510-23

O'Connell, B., Palmer, S., & Williams, H. (2012). *Solution focused coaching in practice*. Routledge. https://doi.org/10.4324/9780203111734

Osmani, M., Weerakkody, V., Hindi, N., & Eldabi, T. (2019). Graduates employability skills: A review of literature against market demand. *Journal of Education for Business*, *94*(7), 423–432. https://doi.org/10.1080/08832323.2018.1545629

Thornton, C. (2016). *Group and team coaching: The secret life of groups* (2nd ed.). Routledge. https://doi.org/10.4324/9781315684956

Tuckman, B. W. (1965). Development sequence in small groups. *Psychological Bulletin*, *63*(6), 384–399. https://doi.org/10.1037/h0022100

Volet, S., & Mansfield, C. (2006). Group work at university: Significance of personal goals in the regulation strategies of students with positive and negative appraisals. *Higher Education Research & Development*, *25*(4), 341–356. https://doi.org/10.1080/07294360600947301

8   Adopting a Coaching Approach to Doctorate Supervision

Rebecca J. Jones

Chapter Objectives

- To discuss the need to reconsider how we supervise doctoral students.
- To define a coaching style of supervision.
- To highlight how supervisors can adopt a coaching approach.

Keywords

coaching
doctoral study
development
supervision

Introduction

As doctoral supervision generally involves one-to-one developmental discussions, it is ideally suited to a coaching approach. Coaching principles can be applied to enhance supervision and consequently improve postgraduate student attainment and satisfaction, as well as raise the student's awareness of their strengths and opportunities for development, encouraging accountability, which is essential for working on an independent piece of research. Coaching skills, techniques and a coaching mindset can be integrated into the stages of doctoral supervision: enculturation, healthy relationships and emancipation to support student outcomes. This chapter will refer to "Supervision", which encompasses predominantly doctoral supervision. However, most of the arguments presented in this chapter can also be applied to master's supervision.

Why Consider Approaches of Supervision?

Doctoral students are susceptible to attrition (Mullen, 2020), with attrition quoted as being as high as 50 per cent (Maddox, 2017). Doloriert et al. (2012) argue that

DOI: 10.4324/9781003332176-10

the process of earning a doctorate is complex, and a critical success factor is the supervisory relationship, with dissatisfaction with the supervisory relationship often cited as a leading cause of these high attrition levels (Maddox, 2017).

Given the importance of the supervisory relationship in the success of doctoral students, it is not surprising that research has focused on the pedagogy of doctoral supervision. Zeegers and Barron (2012) argue that supervision is a blend of pedagogical and personal relationships. However, this relational side needs to be addressed in definitions of doctoral supervision approaches, focusing instead on the knowing supervisor who passes on knowledge to the unknowing student, often linked with master–apprentice metaphors (Bartlett & Mercer, 2001). However, questions have been raised for some time about the applicability of these approaches to doctoral supervision (Bartlett & Mercer, 2001), as such representations of the student ignore the pre-requisites for entering the doctoral programme and the discipline and institutional knowledge that a doctoral student must have to gain candidacy (Zeegers & Barron, 2012).

An alternative approach to doctoral supervision is a coaching approach, which brings the relationship to the fore and influences how supervisors interact with their doctoral students.

Defining Coaching in the Context of Supervision

Coaching is a learning and development tool to produce behavioural change (Jones, 2020). Supervisors who adopt a coaching approach demonstrate a coaching mindset, for example, being open and curious, adopting a non-judgemental attitude (they ask rather than assume) and having a growth mindset (they believe people can learn and change) (Dweck, 2006). They also use coaching behaviours such as listening, goal-setting and creating a reflective space to enable learning from experience. The coachee leads coaching, and the coach and coachee work collaboratively on an equal standing (Jones & Andrews, 2019).

It is important to distinguish between a coach and a supervisor adopting a coaching approach. Supervisors will always be subject-matter experts and provide advice, and there will also be a power difference between the supervisor and doctoral student. Whereas coaches are generally not subject-matter experts, they refrain from giving advice and strive for equal power distribution. The functions of advising, teaching, guiding and directing will always be essential components of supervision, for example, when supporting students in areas where they have very little knowledge. In contrast, these functions rarely form part of a traditional coaching engagement. Despite these differences between coaching and supervision, supervisors and students alike can benefit when supervisors adopt coaching principles.

Some of these benefits have been outlined in the literature. For example, Godskesen and Kobayashi (2015) argue that coaching doctoral students can help students identify and overcome ill-defined problems that may hinder progress in their doctoral study process. Overall et al. (2011) found that doctoral students with supervisors who encourage them to think and act autonomously while still guiding them on research tasks reported higher research self-efficacy, and Nichol et al. (2018) argue that a coaching approach to doctoral supervision results in the transfer and sustainability of learning.

Adopting a coaching approach does not diminish the traditional supervisory role but enhances it. Defining coaching within supervision signifies a shift towards a more dynamic, student-centred approach to doctoral supervision that prioritises the student's own expertise and encourages accountability for academic and personal growth.

A Coaching Approach to Supervision

To outline a coaching approach to supervision grounded in the current supervision literature, I take Gray and Crosta's (2018) components of doctoral supervision (which are based on Lee's (2011) framework, and I blend this framework with coaching principles (Figure 8.1). Gray and Crosta (2018) conducted a systematic literature review of 152 original articles to ascertain doctoral supervision best practices. They suggest that the results can be grouped into three themes: enculturation, healthy relationships and emancipation.

Enculturation

Enculturation is the process of socialising doctoral students into the academic world (Lee, 2011) so that they understand academia and gain a sense of belonging. Gray and Crosta (2018) outline that during the enculturation stage, expectations around how the relationship will work should be managed, and ground rules outlining what each party expects of the other, such as around the provision of feedback, should be agreed (Nichol et al., 2018).

These principles of setting expectations and agreeing on ground rules as part of the enculturation process are closely aligned with the contracting stage of coaching. When coaches contract with their coachees, they are discussing and agreeing (Dotlich & Cairo, 1999):

1 What needs to happen and in what context.
2 They are establishing trust and a set of mutual expectations.
3 They are contracting for results.

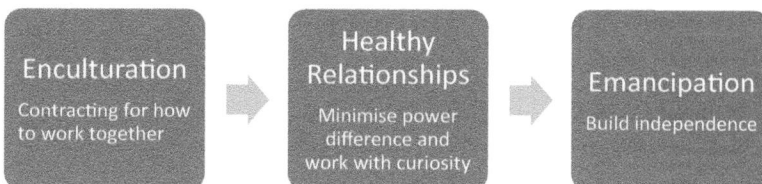

Figure 8.1 The doctoral process

A supervisor adopting a coaching style can equally effectively apply these contracting principles. For example, by discussing and agreeing on what needs to happen and in what context, the supervisor and student will discuss and decide how they will work together (Box 8.1).

If the first step of contracting concerns "what" will happen in supervision (or the process side of supervision), the next step focuses on the relationship side, as the supervisor and student establish trust and a mutual set of expectations. A supportive relationship is essential in effective coaching (Jones & Andrews, 2019), and, equally, the relationship between supervisor and student is integral to effective supervision (Zeegers & Barron, 2012). Multiple factors contribute to an effective, trusting relationship, with the process of contracting itself starting to develop this relationship.

Whether made explicit or not, when entering a working relationship, we enter into a psychological contract, which sets out our expectations and beliefs around our obligations to one another. Trust can be ruptured if we break this psychological contract by not fulfilling these expectations and obligations. We create the solid foundations for a trusting relationship by explicitly discussing and agreeing to our expectations. Foy (2020) argues that we can further solidify this relationship during the contracting stage by discussing the "what ifs". In doctoral supervision, the supervisor and student discuss how to manage "what if" situations. For example, what if we find that we are not getting along? What if the feedback is unclear? What if the two supervisors disagree? Foy (2020) argues that while covering every eventuality is impossible, it is possible to explore a few key areas that can form the basis of a trusting working relationship.

Finally, supervisors can contract with students for results for the enculturation stage. This involves explicitly discussing their motivations and ambitions for the research, which can inform the ongoing supervision relationship. Positioning this conversation around motivations and ambitions after the contracting has taken place means that the supervisor has started to build the

---

Box 8.1 Coaching Questions for Establishing the Ground Rules of Supervision

- How frequently will they meet?
- How long will the meetings be?
- Who will set the agenda for the meetings?
- What will the format of the meetings be (i.e. face to face or online)?
- How should the supervisor and student interact in between meetings?
- How will feedback on written work be managed?
- What will the turnaround time on feedback be?
- If there are multiple supervisors, how will this be managed?
- Which supervisor should the student approach with questions?

required rapport with the student before turning to what may be, for some students, more thought-provoking questions to explore. Once a supportive relationship between supervisor and student has been established, students may be able to openly explore their motivations and ambitions (as well as their fears and reservations) with their supervisor. Coaching questions for this discussion include:

• What motivated you to decide to pursue a PhD?
• What are your goals related to your research?
• What are your plans after your research is complete? How might your research support these plans?

Healthy Relationships

I have already touched on the importance of the trusting relationship between supervisor and student. This relationship is argued to be instrumental to student satisfaction and the completion of studies (Andrew, 2012). Gray and Crosta (2018) suggest that the complex nature of the relationship calls for supervisors to be confident and able to adapt to the inevitable ups and downs students experience while conducting their research. The sense of connection that students experience in a healthy supervisory relationship enables them to be open and receptive and more deeply engaged in learning (Bradbury-Jones et al., 2010). Fundamental to a healthy relationship is trust. Trust develops over time and, therefore, must be continually nurtured so that it endures throughout the relationship, withstanding ruptures that will inevitably occur during disagreements or challenging stages of the research process.

This emphasis on the relationship between supervisor and student closely aligns with a coaching approach to supervision. For example, a coaching approach to supervision emphasises the importance of the supervisor's non-judgemental attitude, which plays a vital role in developing a trusting relationship. If we feel that someone is judging us negatively, we are unlikely to experience intense feelings of trust towards that person. Supervisors who take a coaching approach also adopt a growth mindset (the belief that individuals can grow and develop rather than having fixed abilities) (Dweck, 2006), which also facilitates trust as it links to the issue of judgement. A supervisor with a growth mindset is communicating to their student: I am not passing judgement on the limits of your ability.

As supervisors, we can challenge ourselves to remain non-judgemental during student interactions. This means refraining from hypothesising why a student may have behaved and interacted in a particular way. For example, we may notice that a student always sends us work in draft form, with multiple spelling and grammatical errors. The student needs to proofread their work before sending it for review. However, to remain non-judgemental, we need to challenge ourselves rather than hypothesise such as this. Therefore, as soon as we notice a judgement starting to form, we first notice that the judgement is forming, pause, acknowledge that we are forming a judgement (which is a natural human reaction) and then decide to adopt a stance of curiosity instead. We can adopt a curious stance by asking the student for clarification in an open and non-confrontational way. For example, in the case of the earlier example, you might ask: "I notice that the drafts you share often have some spelling errors in them. I wonder what the reasons for that might be?" Alternatively, if you find that your student is making a point that you disagree with, before arguing for the alternative, you might ask: "That is an interesting perspective. Can you tell me more about your thoughts behind it?" (Box 8.2).

Power

An essential point of acknowledgement about healthy relationships is power. In doctoral supervision, a power imbalance has been argued to be inevitable, and students often feel powerless (Grant, 2003). However, it is vital that supervisors explicitly acknowledge the presence of power in the supervisor–student relationship and that the power dynamics are managed as the student develops to become an independent researcher (Gray & Crosta, 2018).

Conversely to the supervisory relationship, most definitions of coaching emphasise the equal nature of the relationship between the coach and the coachee (Jones & Andrews, 2019). However, this approach is arguably naïve given that power is a central concept in organisations and relationships: Can any relationship between two individuals be devoid of power differences? For example, given the notion that "knowledge is power" and that coaching is intended as a form of knowledge exchange (even if this is through the facilitation of learning rather than direct instruction), it can be argued that the power of the coach is implicit (Garvey & Stokes, 2021). Power will always be present in doctoral supervision, even when a coaching approach to supervision is adopted.

Box 8.2   Principles for Formulating Coaching Questions

- Use open rather than closed questions (i.e. open questions often start with "what" or "how").
- Avoid stacking questions (i.e. asking more than one question at once).
- Avoid hiding advice in a question (i.e. have you thought about …?).
- Avoid providing multiple choice questions (i.e. is it about A or B? It could be about option C, D or E, which we have not even thought of).
- Avoid asking "why?" questions as these can come across as critically questioning judgement (i.e. why did you do that? Can lead to defensiveness). Usually, replacing "why" with phrases such as "I wonder what the reasons are" or "Tell me more about what informed your decision here" can help to keep the thinking open.

However, Like Grant (2003) and Gray and Crosta (2018), I argue that these power dynamics must be explicitly acknowledged and managed to ensure a healthy coaching relationship between supervisor and student. The supervisor will always hold most of the power given their legitimate role. Demonstrating how this power manifests includes the power the supervisor has over when a student is ready for confirmation and when the thesis is ready for submission. Nichol et al. (2018) argues that even when a coaching approach to supervision is adopted, and an aura of equality and mutuality is present, there is still the need to be mindful of the power imbalance, even when working with students who are senior practitioners.

Steps can be taken to address this power imbalance and enable the student to experience greater agency in the supervision process. For example, as detailed in the earlier section on contracting, adopting a student-led approach enables the student to influence ways of working by creating a trusting relationship with high psychological safety where the student can speak up if they disagree with the supervisor. To create a psychologically safe working relationship, supervisors must demonstrate that they are also open to receiving feedback from their students, role modelling an open and curious stance when students speak up, provide feedback or challenge ideas.

Supervisors can also seek to address the power imbalance by always starting with asking questions rather than immediately opting to provide advice. Advice and information sharing will always be integral to effective doctoral supervision. However, supervisors should ask, "What have you considered?", consequently empowering students. There are several additional benefits when supervisors hold back from advising students:

- Students can build their self-evaluation skills by being challenged to explore their solutions.
- Open questions encourage students to reflect and draw on what they already know.
- Helps students prepare for the final element of the doctoral journal: emancipation from the supervisor.

Emancipation

The final stage outlined by Gray and Crosta (2018) is the emancipatory phase, where students become independent or free from their supervisor. Emancipation involves the development of student independence so that they become an autonomous researcher in their own right. When students achieve emancipation, they demonstrate their ability to cope with change, are proactive in deciding their research direction and demonstrate an understanding of the values embedded within the academia (Lee, 2011).

A universal goal of coaching is to enable coachees to take responsibility for their thoughts and actions (Whitmore, 2017), which closely aligns with the independence described in the emancipation stage of supervision. I have already mentioned the importance of asking questions; however, asking questions can also help students to effectively reach the emancipation stage, taking responsibility for their thoughts and actions about their research. When asked a question, it forces us to take responsibility to come to a resolution, providing increased accountability for our actions. A simple way to start this shift from tell to ask is when a student presents a problem, ask them to share their views and ideas before you share yours.

Hand in hand with asking questions is another coaching skill: listening. When someone listens to us, we feel truly heard. It sends the message that we have something worth listening to, something of value. Sending the message to your students that they have something worth listening to helps build their confidence, positioning them as capable, independent researchers rather than "just" students. Supervisors adopting a coaching style truly listen and pay attention to their students. A case study is presented in Box 8.3 that shares the perspective of a doctoral students who was supervised by a supervisor who used a coaching style.

Box 8.3   Case Example

The following case example is provided by Dr Julia Carden whose doctoral research focused on the topic of self-awareness in adult development. Dr Carden provides her perspective as a doctoral student, having been supervised by a supervisor who utilised a coaching style.

As a doctoral student there are times when you want and need clear direction and advice, and other times when you want your thinking challenged in an empathetic, constructive way rather than an adversarial way, this is where your supervisor can make maximum use of a coaching style. Thinking about the Myles Downey (Downey, 2014) spectrum of Directive to Non-Directive coaching it works well when one's supervisor uses the full spectrum of Directive and Non-Directive coaching. I particularly valued a non-directive coaching style when I was floundering, felt lost and wanted a confidence boost, and more directive coaching when I needed a steer in the right direction.

I did my PhD by publication. Initially in working on the draft paper for publication, my supervisor challenged my thinking about the journal I was aiming to publish in by eliciting my expectations; my hopes and aspirations and my understanding of the challenges involved. Once I had done some of my own independent thinking and research into journal options, she then provided some guidance on the journals to aim for. It really resourced me to go and research journal options in the first place and then seek agreement with my supervisor.

In drafting the paper for publication my supervisor proactively asked challenging coaching questions throughout the drafting stage rather than simply giving me direct feedback and this gave me the opportunity to grow as a researcher. Questions like "what was your thinking behind this; and what's the message you are wanting to convey?" really helped me frame and refine my writing style.

There was clear movement between a directive coaching approach, e.g. "have you thought about this?" or, "it would be/might be helpful to think about ..."; to a non-directive approach, e.g. "What are you hoping to achieve with this?", and "what support do you need to complete this paper?"

Throughout the PhD supervision, there was ongoing moral support through using a coaching style, e.g. "How are you progressing?", "How are you feeling?" and "What strengths can you draw on?" This was vital as it helped keep me motivated. It would have been easy for me to seek my supervisor's approval and be given or not given it. While this might have enabled me to produce a PhD, I do not believe I would have grown and developed as much as a researcher and a person as I did, having experienced a coaching style and approach of PhD supervision.

Insights from the case study:

- By using coaching skills to contract at the start of the supervision, the supervisor was able to bring the student back to these original objectives later in the journey by asking the student to reflect on these objectives in the context of addressing dilemmas (such as identifying a target publication)
- The supervisor navigated between providing advice and guidance in areas where the student had little or no knowledge and using open questions to explore the students' views. For example, rather than moving immediately to advising on writing style, ask the student, "What is the message you want to convey?"
- Providing the student with autonomy regarding the direction and content of the supervision sessions demonstrates confidence and trust in the student's ability to manage the process of their studies. For example, asking, "What would you like to focus on today?"
- Using coaching questions to encourage the student to reflect on and draw upon their existing strengths to enable them to move towards independence as a researcher. For example, asking, "What strengths can you draw on to address this challenge?"

Supporting Struggling Students

The three stages of the doctoral process described in this chapter (enculturation, healthy relationships, emancipation) only partially account for some of the challenges students may encounter. The doctorate process is, by definition, a long, drawn-out process with extended periods where the student must work independently with sporadic deadlines. Successful completion relies on excellent time management, project management and organisational skills. It is common for students to lose momentum, experience doubts in confidence, struggle with focus, find it challenging to take onboard feedback or become overwhelmed with the scale of the project. Coaching can be a useful tool for students struggling with any of these issues at the supervisor's disposal to support them. Table 8.1 shows potential coaching solutions for some common challenges doctoral students encounter.

Table 8.1 Coaching Solutions for Common Doctoral Student Challenges

Challenge	Coaching solution	Further information
Loss of momentum	Exploration of values	To persist with a challenging goal, we need to see how this links to the bigger picture. Working with the student's values can support this. Using a values framework such as Schwartz (1994), ask the student to reflect on: • Which value(s) resonate with you? • Which values are most important and what are the reasons for this? • How would you describe the link between your values and your decision to pursue a doctorate?
Doubts in confidence	Letter from the future[a]	Ask your student to imagine a point in the future when they have successfully completed their doctorate. Their task is to write a letter to themselves now from their future self. What would this future self (who has achieved the doctorate) say to them now? How does it feel to achieve this goal? What have they learnt along the way? Encourage the student to be as specific and detailed as possible. They should keep the letter in an envelope to read again. Ask the student to reflect on the process of writing the letter: what insights did they gain?
Struggle with focus	2 × 2 matrix[a]	A 2 × 2 matrix enables students to map and prioritise different options. This may be helpful for students who are struggling to focus due to competing demands. The students should decide what criterion they will use on each axis of the 2 × 2 grid (i.e. urgent vs important, impact vs ease of action, etc.). Once the axes are labelled, the student can now identify all various activities or options available to them and place these in the relevant quadrant. Once this is complete, the student can step back to review the results. Ask the student: what is this telling you about your next steps?

(Continued)

Table 8.1 (Continued)

Challenge	Coaching solution	Further information
Responding to feedback	Cognitive behavioural coaching	There are many reasons why individuals may struggle to respond to feedback. One reason may involve taking feedback very personally. Cognitive behavioural coaching may be a useful technique to support students in overcoming this challenge. Cognitive behavioural coaching involves supporting the coachee to identify, challenge and generate alternative thoughts, attitudes and beliefs (Willson, 2020). A relatively simple way of exploring this with a student is with the following questions: • What script are you telling yourself in relation to this feedback? • How is this script helping you to move on with this piece of work? • How might you rewrite your script in a way which is aligned with your broader goal?
Becoming overwhelmed	Gantt chart	The most effective course of action to reduce overwhelm is to create a detailed action plan. A tool such as a Gantt chart can be useful to help the student breakdown and organise the full range of tasks that need to be completed. These tasks should be as detailed as possible. For example, listing "complete literature review" is not helpful in reducing overwhelm. Ask the student to break every task into the smallest sub-task possible. Each sub-task can then be allocated a deadline. This detailed approach to planning will not only help with reducing overwhelm, it will also support the supervisor in monitoring progress and help the student maintain momentum.

[a] For further information see Flower (2020).

Conclusion

Often, very little guidance or support is provided to supervisors beyond informing them of their intuitions, policies and procedures. Indeed, being a subject matter expert with a PhD is often assumed to equip the individual with everything they need to supervise others. This may be why supervisors often default to the style of supervision they received from their supervisors when they were students. The statistics demonstrate that attrition of doctoral students is an issue and that the supervisors' role is pivotal in the success and satisfaction of students. Therefore, a coaching approach to doctoral supervision may solve these challenges. In this chapter, I have defined a coaching approach to supervision and illustrated how we might integrate coaching with the supervision process. Supervisors may benefit from attending coaching skills training to deepen their knowledge of coaching and enable them to practice and develop coaching skills. Due to the unique nature of the supervisor–student relationship, specifically the inherent power imbalance and requirement for the supervisor to share knowledge with the student, supervisors will never be "true" coaches when in their role as doctoral supervisors. However, this is not to say that a blended approach of traditional supervision with a coaching style cannot work well throughout all stages of the supervisory process.

Coaching Questions

- What are your expectations for this supervisory relationship?
- How do you think you could overcome this problem?
- How are you going to organise your time?
- What strengths do you have that will help you in completing your research?
- What do you anticipate will be the most significant challenges?
- What might be the reason why you are feeling stuck writing this chapter?
- What do you think?
- What alternative theories/methods might work here?
- How would you articulate your contribution to someone you met in the street?
- What do you think an examiner might focus on in your defence?

What questions in your defence are you most concerned about answering, and why do you think that is the case?

Summary

- Traditional conceptualisations of doctoral supervision often link to the master–apprentice metaphor, do not acknowledge the resources within students and under-emphasise the relational aspects of supervision.
- A coaching approach to supervision is student-led, places importance on the trusting relationship and encourages using coaching skills during supervisory meetings.
- Power imbalance will always be present in supervision. However, coaching can help to mitigate and manage this imbalance.
- A coaching approach to supervision can be considered at three stages of the supervisory process:

  - Enculturation – the process of socialising the student into the academic world. Utilising the principle of contracting from coaching will facilitate effective enculturation.
  - Healthy relationships – the ongoing healthy, trusting relationship between supervisor and student. Adopting principles from coaching can assist in forming and maintaining a healthy relationship, specifically a non-judgemental attitude and growth mindset.

- Emancipation – the development of student independence. The coaching skills of asking questions and listening will facilitate responsibility-taking and foster the growth of self-belief.

Discussion Starters

- How would you define your supervisory style?
- How would your students describe your supervisory style?
- How do you structure your first supervisory session with students?
- How can you incorporate the suggestions from the enculturation/contracting stage detailed in this chapter in your supervision?
- What kind of questions do you ask your students?
- How do you indicate to your students that you are genuinely listening?
- What actions do you take that facilitate a trusting relationship with students?

References

Andrew, M. (2012). Supervising doctorates at a distance: Three trans-tasman stories. *Quality Assurance in Education, 20*(1), 42–53. https://doi.org/10.1108/096848812 11198239

Bartlett, A., & Mercer, G. (2001). Introduction. In A. Bartlett & G. Mercer (Eds), *Postgraduate research supervision: Transforming (r)elations* (pp. 1–5), Peter Lang Publishing.

Bradbury-Jones, C., Irvine, F., & Sambrook, S. (2010). Empowerment of nursing students in clinical practice: Spheres of influence. *Journal of Advanced Nursing, 66*(9), 2061–2070. https://doi.org/10.1111/j.1365-2648.2010.05351.x

Doloriert, C., Sambrook, S., & Stewart, J. (2012). Power and emotion in doctoral supervision: Implications for HRD. *European Journal of Training and Development, 36*(7), 732–750. https://doi.org/10.1108/03090591211255566

Dotlich, D. L., & Cairo, P. C. (1999). *Action coaching: How to leverage individual performance for company success.* Jossey-Bass.

Downey, M. (2014). *Effective modern coaching.* LID Publishing.

Dweck, C. (2006). *Mindset: The new psychology of success.* Random House.

Flower, J. (2020). Fifteen tools and techniques for coaches. In J. Passmore (Ed.), *The coaches' handbook* (pp. 427–442). Routledge. https://doi.org/10.4324/978100308988 9-46

Foy, K. (2020). Contracting in coaching. In J. Passmore (Ed.), *The coaches' handbook* (pp. 344–354). Routledge. https://doi.org/10.4324/9781003089889-37

Garvey, R., & Stokes, P. (2021). *Coaching and mentoring: Theory and practice* (4th ed.). SAGE Publications.

Godskesen, M., & Kobayashi, S. (2015). Coaching doctoral students – A means to enhance progress and support self-organisation in doctoral education. *Studies in Continuing Education, 38*(2), 145–161. https://doi.org/10.1080/0158037x.2015.1055464

Grant, B. (2003). Mapping the pleasures and risks of supervision. *Discourse: Studies in the Cultural Politics of Education, 24*(2), 175–190. https://doi.org/10.1080/01596300 303042

Gray, M. A., & Crosta, L. (2018). New perspectives in online doctoral supervision: A systematic literature review. *Studies in Continuing Education, 41*(2), 173–190. https://doi.org/10.1080/0158037x.2018.1532405

Jones, R. J. (2020). *Coaching with research in mind.* Routledge. https://doi.org/10.4324/9780429431746

Jones, R. J., & Andrews, H. (2019). Understanding the rise of faculty–student coaching: An academic capitalism perspective. *Academy of Management Learning & Education*, *18*(4), 606–625. https://doi.org/10.5465/amle.2017.0200

Lee, A. (2011). *Successful research supervision*. Routledge. https://doi.org/10.4324/978020 3816844

Maddox, S. (2017). *Did not finish: Doctoral attrition in higher education and student affairs* [Doctoral thesis, University of Northern Colorado]. Scholarship & Creative Works @ Digital UNC. https://digscholarship.unco.edu/dissertations/433/

Mullen, C. A. (2020). Online doctoral mentoring in a pandemic: Help or hindrance to academic progress on dissertations? *International Journal of Mentoring and Coaching in Education*, 10(2), 139–157. https://doi.org/10.1108/ijmce-06-2020-0029

Nichol, L., Cook, J., & Ross, C. (2018). Adopting coaching for doctoral supervision: Opportunities and challenges for HRD. *Human Resource Development International*, *25*(4), 488–499. https://doi.org/10.1080/13678868.2018.1547038

Overall, N. C., Deane, K. L., & Peterson, E. R. (2011). Promoting doctoral students' research self-efficacy: Combining academic guidance with autonomy support. *Higher Education Research & Development*, *30*(6), 791–805. https://doi.org/10.1080/0729436 0.2010.535508

Schwartz, S. H. (1994). Beyond individualism/collectivism: New cultural dimensions of values. In U. Kim, H. C. Triandis, Ç. Kâğitçibaşi, S. C. Choi, & G. Yoon (Eds), *Individualism and collectivism: Theory, method, and applications* (pp. 85–119). SAGE Publications.

Whitmore, J. (2017). *Coaching for performance: The principles and practice of coaching and leadership*. Nicholas Brealey Publishing.

Willson, R. (2020). Cognitive-behavioural coaching. In J. Passmore (Ed.), *The coaches' handbook* (pp. 208 – 220), Routledge. https://doi.org/10.4324/9781003089889-24

Zeegers, M., & Barron, D. (2012). Pedagogical concerns in doctoral supervision: A challenge for pedagogy. *Quality Assurance in Education*, *20*(1), 20–30. https://doi.org/10.1108/09684881211198211

Part III

Coaching To Prepare the Future Workforce

9 Coaching for Workplace Internships

Is My Coachee a Student or an Employee?

Peng Cheng Wang, Rendell Kheng Wah Tan, May Sok Mui Lim and Chee Ming Ong

---

Chapter Objectives

- To provide an overview of work-based learning in higher education and the role of academic supervisors as coaches.
- To highlight various opportunities to coach for developing transferable skills and a growth mindset.
- To discuss the application of the GROW model for workplace coaching.
- To explore the development of critical thinking skills through journaling.
- To identify coachable moments and "not to coach" areas.
- To evaluate the implementation of coaching at a programme level.

Keywords

academic supervisor
coaching conversations
coachable moments
internship
journalling
reframing
transferable skills
workplace learning
workplace supervisor

Introduction

Workplace learning, also called work-based learning or internship, is becoming increasingly important for students to relate the acquired knowledge to its application in a workplace environment. This allows students to develop holistically in both technical and professional skills. Workplace learning can be

DOI: 10.4324/9781003332176-12

realised during a student's internship with an organisation, where there will be expectations to simultaneously manage the responsibilities of being a student and an employee. University academic supervisors, therefore, play a pivotal role in coaching their students towards deepening their specialist skills to spur students to apply what they have learnt in the university at the workplace, ensuring good integration of work and study. Coaching at this juncture is critical as supervisors empower and encourage students to take on a growth mindset of self-directed progress to develop a workplace spirit of excellence. Professional traits identified by the World Economic Forum (2023) for career success in the twenty-first century, such as adaptability, ability to work with people, effective communications and critical thinking, are areas where the students can be coached for better internship performance at the workplace and after graduation. When an issue arises, instead of merely focusing on solving the immediate problem, university supervisors can use this opportunity as a coachable moment to coach their students to explore the challenge, work on finding solutions and take ownership for actions that can progressively propel them towards achieving their goals. In other words, coach the person, not the problem.

Coaching benefits all students, including those who are doing well and are motivated to develop themselves to be excellent performers at work. This chapter will look beyond just the 1:1 coaching relationship between the educator and student. We will extend the discussion to include the workplace supervisor's perspectives on getting students to consider the organisation's practices and culture, the nature of the work, and the reality of working with bosses, peers and subordinates. We will discuss the Feldman Tripartite model (Feldmann, 2016) and highlight case studies to show the effectiveness of workplace coaching during internships.

Workplace Learning in Higher Education

Undergraduate internships are increasingly gaining importance and emphasised across degree programmes (Goller et al., 2020; Peters et al., 2019). This integration of internships into the curriculum is a paradigm shift, from seeing students as workers who are learning to work, to students as learners who are working on learning (Luk & Chan, 2021). The need to interrelate knowledge acquired in class to its application in the work environment is gaining attention, especially with the growing emphasis on concurrently developing both technical and professional skills (Bayerlein, 2020; Maaravi et al., 2020). Findings from more recent literature highlight the positive benefits of internship, such as increased student motivation in their degree choice and invaluable industry connections (Goller et al., 2020). Done correctly, where the relevant internship experience is contextualised in an actual workplace environment, students are able to appreciate the expectations and challenges in their eventual chosen profession (Bayerlein, 2020). Students can also develop specific professional competencies in their chosen field, leading to professional advancement and to cope with future job demands (Goller et al., 2020).

Role of Academic Supervisors as Coaches

Coaching is increasingly used in education to build students' emotional resilience and to improve their performance, goal attainment and workplace well-being (Schroth, 2019; Tee et al., 2019). Feldmann (2016) proposed a tripartite framework to describe the roles played by the university, the industry partner, and the student. Figure 9.1 shows an adaptation of Feldmann's model of coaching in the context of workplace learning.

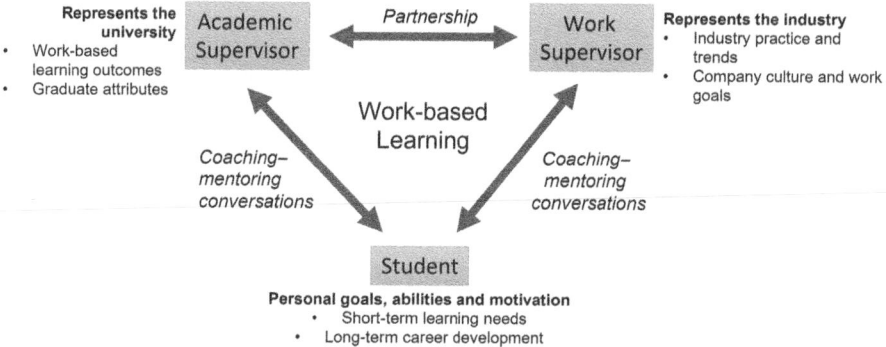

Figure 9.1 Adaptation of Feldmann's Tripartite model in the context of coaching

In the workplace, coaching helps students build their social capital and have role models (Molyn, 2020) they can look up to and seek guidance and advice. When viewed from a coaching perspective, the framework highlights the parallel coaching conversations between the student and the work supervisor, and between the student and the academic supervisor. As the work supervisor, academic supervisor and student represent different perspectives, the partnership between the industry work supervisor and the university academic supervisor completes the tripartite relationship and make workplace learning successful.

Schroth (2019) suggests that more is expected of workplace supervisors where the students value 1:1, collaborative and reflective relationships. This means that for such relationships to be effective, purposeful feedback through coaching conversations is essential for the students to develop, grow and achieve the desired competence. This integration of coaching with timely and calibrated feedback is critical for developing the students in their workplace. Aligning students' and supervisors' expectations can also increase collaboration (Peters et al., 2019). In work-based learning, the academic supervisor and work supervisor assume the role of coaches, with the student as the coachee. The coach-coachee relationship needs to be built on mutual trust and respect, and is the critical enabler for the coachees to be receptive to feedback (Atkinson et al., 2021).

While on placement, students are expected to manage the responsibilities of being a student and an employee simultaneously. The university academic supervisor plays a pivotal role in coaching their students towards deepening their specialist skills and ensuring good integration of work and study. This goes beyond traditional academic advising, with the combined academic-industry focus enabling students to reflect and develop their early career plans (Molyn, 2020; Tudor, 2018). Coaching at this juncture is, therefore, of critical significance. Academic supervisors can empower and encourage students to develop a growth mindset for self-directed progress and a spirit of excellence at the workplace. This excellence cannot just be defined narrowly within the confines of being good at the required specialised skill sets but also the ability to adapt, perform and thrive in the workplace environment. In this respect, the academic supervisor can partner with the work supervisor to meet the student's short-term learning needs and longer-term career development. Subsequent discussions for the rest of this chapter will focus primarily on the academic supervisor as the coach.

Coaching to Develop Students' Transferable Skills

To prepare students for the world of work, it is important to recognise the value of transferable skills to complement the in-depth technical training that the university provides. While there can be various means to develop these transferable skills in university students, internships provide the most authentic environment for students to acquire these skills (Feldmann, 2016). The literature reviewed in this chapter on workplace learning suggests that most studies use the theoretical lens of experiential learning theory to show that when students are placed in real-world situations in the workplace, they have to practise these skills and be competent in them. The nature of workplace learning is more complex compared to classroom learning, which tends to be organised and guided. Learning at the workplace tends to be less structured as it involves both formal and informal learning (Luk & Chan, 2021). The success of workplace learning strongly correlates to job satisfaction, and more critically, good industry supervision and support contributed equally significantly to job satisfaction (Maaravi et al., 2020).

The professional traits for career success such as adaptability, ability to work with people, communication effectively and critical thinking, are areas the students can be coached on for better work performance. These are essential life skills that tertiary students will need in their workplace – during an internship and when they graduate (Cronin et al., 2019). When a workplace challenge arises, it presents a good coachable moment for the supervisors to have a coaching conversation with the student, not just for solving the immediate problem but also to coach the student holistically and empower him to take ownership for action towards his goals.

Coaching for a Growth Mindset

A growth mindset is a belief that human attributes are malleable and can be developed (Dweck, 2006). It can affect an individual's self-regulation, resilience, and challenge-seeking tendencies (Dweck & Leggett, 1988; Dweck, 2006). In a study by Ng et al. (2020), students with a growth mindset received better ratings from their work supervisors in problem-solving and decision-making at the end of their workplace internship. This study highlights the imperative of having a growth mindset, such that these individuals are more open to challenges and experimentation in their pursuit of achieving their goals. The study suggests the importance for academic and work supervisors to use a coaching approach with their students instead of offering immediate or direct solutions. With the focus on coaching to develop a growth mindset at the workplace, students can discover their own capabilities and work towards raising their self-efficacy and belief in their learning capacity to achieve their goal.

To coach for developing a growth mindset, the supervisor needs to help students reframe their challenges as opportunities for learning and growth. When students meet their university academic supervisor to ask for help in overcoming a challenge, the supervisor should see this as a coachable moment, asking them to reflect on their strengths and past experiences in successful problem-solving, which can help them find solutions for their current challenge. The students can develop self-belief and confidence that even in the face of a difficult situation, they have the underlying capabilities to overcome it. In the first vignette in Box 9.1, we show how supervisors can coach students in identifying the skills they need to work on, the knowledge they need to learn and strategies to consider when overcoming a challenge.

Box 9.1   Coach for Growth Mindset

Professor Williams sat across the table from her student, Sarah, who was interning with a local IT company. Sarah looked tired and deflated. She had been working under a workplace supervisor who she felt was making her life miserable.

Sarah:	He is constantly criticising my work, even when it's done well. I can't seem to do anything right in his eyes.
Prof:	(*listened empathetically*) It sounds like your supervisor has very high expectations for your work. What do you think could be the reasons?
Sarah:	(*shrugged*) I'm not sure. Maybe he's just a difficult person.
Prof:	(*smiled*) Perhaps. What other possible reasons?
Sarah:	Maybe he is highly stressed and under pressure?
Prof:	Possible. What else?
Sarah:	(*considers other reasons*) Maybe he wants to push me to a level I am not yet performing.
Prof:	Interesting perspective too, and very plausible. We don't really know, do we? What is the best way to find out?

Sarah:	I can't just ask him why he is being so difficult with me.
Prof:	True. How else can you phrase the question then?
Sarah:	(*thinks for a moment*) Perhaps I can speak to him and ask him to share more about his expectations, but I'm afraid it will make things worse.
Prof:	(*leans forward*) Sometimes, the most challenging conversations are the most important ones. It takes courage to start the conversation, but it's necessary for growth and change. (*Sarah nodded thoughtfully.*)
Prof:	What have you noticed about the company's culture? For example, the pace, how tolerable are they to mistakes, and the type of expectations set across the board?
Sarah:	Hmmm … now that you mentioned it, I recall that they are pretty open in pointing out each other's mistakes in meetings. The company is very fast-paced, and the staff pride themselves in meeting the customer's expectations to the highest standard.
Prof:	That sounds like a good observation you have made there. How might that relate to what you said earlier about your supervisor?
Sarah:	Perhaps, it is quite common that mistakes are being pointed out. And the high expectations are for everyone, including my supervisor?
Prof:	What can you do to find out?
Sarah:	I will find a time to talk to him about the general expectations and what I can do to improve.

Over the next few days, Sarah prepared for the conversation with her supervisor. She practised what she would say and how she would say it. When the day finally came, she was nervous but determined.

To her surprise, the conversation went better than she expected. Her supervisor listened to her concerns and explained that his high expectations would spur his interns to do better. He mentioned the things he was impressed with about Sarah's work and encouraged her to do even better.

Sarah was grateful for the coaching and encouragement from Professor Williams. She realised that she could see things from the work supervisor's point of view, better understand the company's culture and that the difficult situations she faced were opportunities for her to grow. This helped her further develop her growth mindset in seeing mistakes and criticism as opportunities for growth and development.

As Sarah's internship ended, she reflected on the lessons she had learned. She was grateful for her difficult experiences because they taught her the importance of seeing them as challenges to overcome and taking the courage to communicate her feelings. And she knew that she would carry these lessons with her throughout her career.

From the vignette, we can gather a few insights. First, ask questions to help the student to reframe and see things from another perspective, such as plausible reasons for the supervisor to behave in a certain way, what colleagues say or what a peer would do in this situation. Second, focus on what the student can do rather than what cannot be controlled. In this example, Sarah realised she could do something about understanding the supervisor's expectations by talking to him. Third, workplace learning through internships provides opportunities for developing transferable skills and a growth mindset. In this example, Sarah had to develop confidence to start a difficult conversation with her work supervisor. As a possible follow-up coaching conversation, Professor Williams could ask questions to probe how Sarah could begin such a conversation, perhaps in an informal setting with the work supervisor.

Whether the outcome is positive or otherwise, it would be a good learning opportunity when the student can reflect on the lessons learnt. As a coach, we can facilitate such conversations with our students for their work. As academic supervisors, we can have a separate communication channel with the work supervisor to discuss how the student has performed at the workplace. Such collaborations can pave the way for the work supervisor to be also involved in coaching the students.

GROW Model

The GROW model is a popular coaching technique used by coaches in conversations with coachees for problem-solving, goal setting and performance improvement (Whitmore, 2017). Academic supervisors can employ the GROW framework (see Table 9.1) to coach their students during the work attachment.

Table 9.1 GROW Model

G-R-O-W Steps	To Enable Students To
Goals	• Identify and decide the learning and performance goals to develop
Reality	• Assess their current situation when setting their learning and performance goals • See things the way they currently are
Options	• Draw out range of options available towards the identified learning and performance goals
Way Forward	• Make a decision on actions to take • Commit to closing the gaps between current reality and desired performance.

One way to make the internship experience impactful is to incorporate a coaching framework into the internship programme. Such an approach is more systematic and can provide opportunities for all students to reflect and supervisors to coach, rather than wait for students to come forward with an issue they would like to address. Such reflective practices can be incorporated into work-based learning programmes through a journalling process as discussed in the next section.

Critical Reflection through Journalling

Reflection is integral to feedback for three reasons. First, encouraging reflective practice inspires students to think critically about how the feedback from the supervisor (as coach) pertains to them and how they might use it for improvement. Second, reflection on feedback can stimulate informed self-assessment, for instance, thinking critically about how they have performed and the new information the feedback provides about their performance. Finally, fostering reflection on feedback can promote the development of ongoing self-appraisal or self-monitoring skills. In other words, it can teach the student the self-analytical process required for lifelong learning (Sargeant et al., 2008).

In the study by Krackov et al. (2017), reflection on one's actions and feedback is a lifelong learning skill that can long serve the graduate to continually build self-awareness and strive for continuous improvement in professional traits essential to the industry he is in. This is illustrated in Figure 9.2. As students are better informed from the feedback, they can be more focused and intentional in identifying the traits they want to work on or strengthen. The

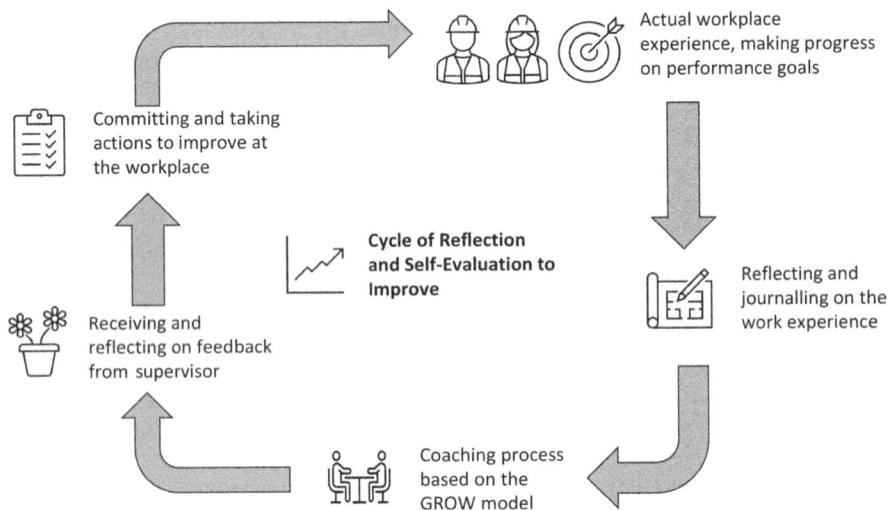

Figure 9.2 Feedback, reflection and coaching

Note: Adapted from "Feedback, reflection and coaching: a new model," by S. K. Krackov, H. S. Pohl, A. S. Peters, and J. M. Sargeant, in J. A. Dent, R. M. Harden, and D. Hunt (Eds), *A practical guide for medical teachers* (5th ed., pp. 287), 2017, Elsevier.

cycle of evaluation and reflection is made possible and gives an added impetus for students to commit to their goals and to achieve them.

The study by Luthans & Peterson (2003) found that one way to improve the effectiveness and impact of feedback for learning and development is to have "360 degrees feedback" (henceforth referred to as 360 feedback) from supervisors (academic and industry), colleagues and peers is to combine them with coaching focused on enhanced self-awareness and behavioural management. Figure 9.3 illustrates the concept.

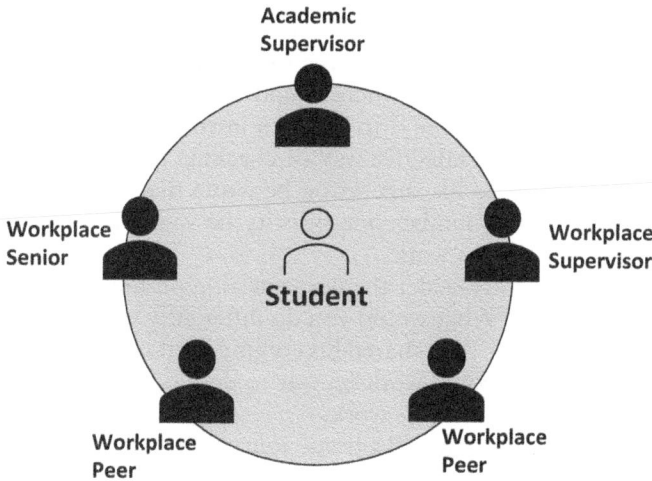

Figure 9.3 360-degree feedback to student during internship

On a regular basis, students can reflect on their workplace performance through the 360 feedback they receive from supervisors, colleagues and peers. This is important as students now have multiple perspectives and sources of information on how they are doing and can reflect on. They will then be able to better identify and commit to improvements in their professional traits, encouraged by the affirmation of the 360 feedback.

In Box 9.2, we give an example of encouraging critical reflection through journalling with coaching questions from the academic supervisor. As you read through the written exchanges between the student and supervisor, there is an intent from the supervisor to encourage the student to find ways to reach his desired goals. The progress is also tracked across the internship period.

In this coaching example, scaling questions were being used to help the student evaluate his current level of achievement as well as set a goal for the internship. The coaching questions act as guides to help students reflect in their journalling process. Scaling is often used in solution-focused coaching to facilitate the coachee in discovering the detailed steps needed to move up the scale to a desired level of achievement. In this case, it was also a way for students to reflect and monitor progress.

Box 9.2   Encouraging Critical Reflection through Journalling with Coaching Questions

Questions based on the GROW coaching model were posed by the academic supervisor Dr Ang to Student Ken.

In the first month of an internship for Accountancy, Ken is required to reflect "On the trait(s) you like to develop, on a scale of 1 (poor) to 10 (excellent), where do you rate yourself now on this trait?" In the first monthly journal report, Ken identified "Care and Diligence" as one of the professional traits that he wishes to develop during the internship programme.

Building on this identified trait, Ken then responded to the next question "On this scale (1 to 10), where would you like to progress to?" He rated himself 6, on a scale of 1 to 10, with intention to move to 8, as he was unsure of the most effective way of checking for mistakes. In Ken's first reflection report to his supervisor, he wrote that he regarded "Care and Diligence" as the number one priority he wants to work on as he tends to rush through his work.

Ken then moves to consider the next question on this reflection-based coaching approach, "What would you do differently to move up a notch on this scale of 1 to 10?" He shared his commitment to improve and identified that an area he could work on was to develop a protocol for error checking before he submits his work.

In the ensuing monthly reflections, journalling his experiences, and commitment actions to improve guided by the coaching questions, Ken was constantly encouraged by Dr Ang on the small wins. Ken felt accountable to his supervisor, given the monthly actions he has committed towards improving his professional trait. He felt empowered as he experienced progress towards his goal of improving his ability to pay attention to details and check for errors.

Five months later …

On Ken's reflections report to Dr Ang, he reported that he improved his "Care and Diligence" trait from 6.0 to 7.5 (scale of 1 to 10). He affirmed that he now has a higher awareness of being careful and not rushing through his work, and is more confident in working towards his intended goal of 8 on the scale. On the commitment question of "Way Forward: Summarise the actions you are committed to take to achieve your goal", Ken journalled that he would continue to "strive to pay attention to details and find different strategies to check for errors especially when given new work conditions".

In Ken's final report in fulfilment of the internship's learning objectives, he acknowledged the importance of professional traits development. He also shared his gratitude and appreciation for his supervisor's moral support and guidance towards his learning success and professional growth.

Case Study of Embedding Coaching into a University's Work-Based Learning Programme

The following is a case study at Singapore Institute of Technology (SIT) of how coaching can be embedded into a university course at the programme level. In this case, the GROW model (Whitmore, 2017) was used to structure the coaching while students were encouraged to reflect critically through journaling.

The Bachelor of Engineering with Honours in Aircraft Systems Engineering (ASE) is a three-year direct honours programme developed in collaboration with Singapore International Airlines Engineering Company (SIAEC), which provides extensive Maintenance, Repair and Overhaul (MRO) services to more than 80 international airlines and aerospace equipment manufacturers worldwide (Singapore Institute of Technology, n.d.). Built on an interdisciplinary curriculum that intersects engineering and science, the programme adopts a practical, hands-on approach to produce theoretically grounded and practice-oriented graduates for the aerospace and MRO industries. This is enabled through the internship programme, where the learning outcomes mainly focus on acquiring technical knowledge and skills in aircraft maintenance. The ASE academic supervisory team decided to enhance the learning experience of their students in developing professional traits essential to the aerospace industry through coaching.

Green et al. (2010) studied how a formal internship affects students' perception of traits that employers consider when hiring. They found that students perceive the importance of these traits differently from those of employers. Employers tend to see many traits as equally important, while students have more distinctive views and values of the same traits (i.e. what is more important or relatable to them at a particular time point during the internship). By knowing the traits valued by potential employers, SIT supervisors can better coach students' transitions from academic studies to professional careers during their internship.

The professional traits are values identified by major potential employer-aviation companies, such as SIA Engineering Company, ST Engineering Aerospace, Rolls-Royce, Pratt & Whitney and General Electric. These professional traits (as shown in Table 9.2) in the aviation industry are deemed critical career success factors and hence are important professional foundations for future graduates.

Before their work attachments, ASE students are briefed on professional traits identified by the aerospace companies that are expected of them at the workplace, and that adopting a growth mindset is important for achieving successful learning outcomes.

Students are to decide on the development of one or two professional traits at any one time. Students are asked to reflect and journal monthly on how they are doing on these selected professional traits during their workplace attachments. This reflection and journalling of the professional traits is in addition to their reports every two weeks on their knowledge and work experience gained.

Table 9.2 Identified Professional Traits from Major Aviation Companies

Seven professional traits of an aircraft engineer	
Pursuit of excellence	I strive for the highest professional standards required in my work and aim for the best in all I do.
Safety first	I regard and practise safety as an essential part of my work, maintaining and adopting practices that promote the safety of airline passengers and colleagues/staff.
Integrity	I set to achieve the highest ethical standards and professionalism, always fully accountable to myself, the organisation and society.
Teamwork	I work cohesively, adding value to the team, working with pride to achieve success together.
Adaptability	I am able to learn, unlearn and relearn, embracing change and adapting to demands at the workplace.
Problem solving	I am a Thinking Tinkerer, passionate in my work, able to apply the knowledge learned, and constantly looking to improve and solve problems.
Effective communications	I listen to understand, am empathetic, and communicate with clarity and confidence.

In their face-to-face coaching sessions, the academic supervisor will begin by asking the students what they want to achieve, i.e. their performance goals. As they reflect on how they are doing regarding the different professional traits, the students journal the state of where they are for each trait. A guide on a scale of 1 to 10, with 1 being poor and 10 being excellent, provides a broad guide on their self-evaluation. By deciding where they are on this scale, the students reflect and describe their current state in their reports to their academic supervisors.

In alignment with the students journaling their reflection and self-evaluation of their professional traits, we adapted the GROW model sequence to R-G-O-W instead (see Table 9.3). Students' reflection of their current REALITY will challenge them to decide their progressive effort next and commitment to moving one or two notches up the scale (1 to 10) towards their GOAL. Students learned that setting aside time to reflect critically and review their professional traits at work will bring more clarity and focus on their potential gaps for improvement. Guided by the open questions adapted by the academic supervisory team, students are empowered to journal their progress, identify gaps and commit to positive actions to improve. This commitment to improving is further reinforced when students journal and share their self-evaluation and developmental action plans with their respective SIT supervisors.

SIT academic supervisors also play the role of coaches by reading and analysing their assigned students' reflections on professional traits development and progress. Based on the reflections detailed by the students, the SIT supervisors will provide tailored feedback and encouragement to reinforce the

Table 9.3 Reflective Journalling in the Aircraft Systems Engineering Programme

Guiding questions for reflective journalling (adapted from the GROW model)	
Reality	• Among the development traits of an aircraft engineer, what is going on well for you? • What have you done to do well to further this trait? • On the trait you like to develop, on a scale of 1 (poor) to 10 (excellent), where do you rate yourself currently on achieving this trait?
Goal	• On this scale (1 to 10), where would you like to progress to? • Describe what it would be like for you when you achieve this level on the scale. • How would this trait benefit you as an aircraft engineer?
Options	• What would you do differently to move this a notch up on the scale? • What support or resources do you need to help you progress?
Way forward	• Summarise the actions you are committed to take to achieve your goal. • How would you keep track of your progress?

students' commitment to deepen their development and empower the students to internalise the growth of their professional traits.

As part of evaluating this initiative, two cohort of students (graduating classes of 2021 and 2022) have since gone through this exercise and were asked to self-appraise the seven professional traits on where they are before and after their internship programme. The survey results of the 2021 cohort were very encouraging. As seen from Figure 9.4, there is a general trend of improvement in the seven professional traits. All students experienced improvement based on their self-scoring evaluation (before and after internship) in all seven

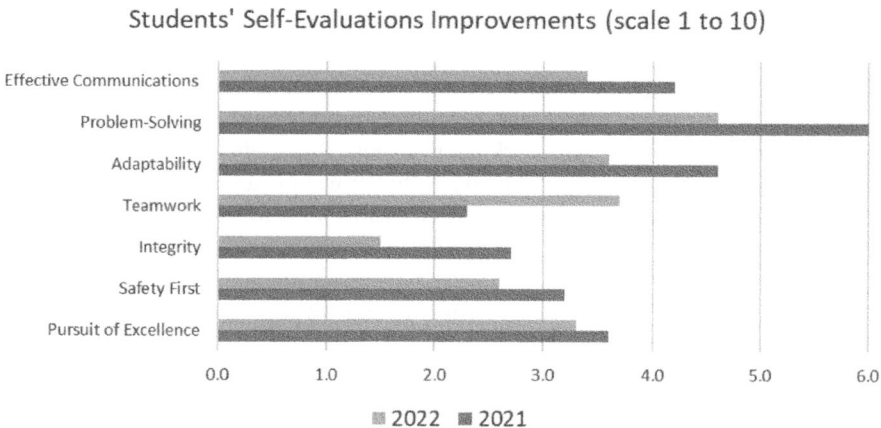

Students' Self-Evaluations Improvements (scale 1 to 10)

Figure 9.4 Professional traits improvements based on students' self-evaluations (2022 and 2021 cohorts)

professional traits. They also shared that the reflections and awareness of the need to self-evaluate and, more importantly, to develop the identified professional traits were beneficial.

The benefits of incorporating the coaching framework at a programmatic level is consistency among different academic supervisors. This ensures that all students in the same programme can be guided in a similar way to reflect. Besides having 1:1 coaching session with students, incorporating regular journalling allows students an extended time to reflect. The university academic supervisor can leverage the student's monthly journal updates to coach and empower the student to achieve his professional goals. Careful nudging to challenge the students to stretch their goals, acknowledge their gradual achievements through the scaffolding enabled by the GROW model and provide encouragement to the students will enhance the impact of the coaching.

For future workplace supervision, the ASE team is exploring the implementation of 360 feedback more comprehensively for more effective coaching of students while they are in the industry during workplace internships. The feedback would include the perspectives of industry supervisor and the peers they work with daily. Industry supervisors' feedback will provide a different perspective for reflection. Questions from industry supervisors may typically come from work-related issues; for example, work culture, different industry supervisors' styles, needs and expectations, and business needs at the point of time. This will vary and usually be quite fluid depending on the circumstances yet offer authenticity in the questions raised. Peer-to-peer feedback is equally important, as peer appraisal can allow students to learn how one's performance will affect another and the team's dynamics. These are valuable learning points for the students as they realise that teamwork in school will vastly differ from teamwork in the workplace. The 360 feedback can provide an all-round holistic evaluation, which will be necessary for students to develop and grow professionally beyond their technical competency.

Conclusion

This chapter has demonstrated the need for a good coaching framework to guide students through their internships while preparing them to be workforce ready. When first exposed, the work environment is usually unique, foreign and overwhelming to the students. Yet, these challenges present valuable opportunities for coaching students so that they can learn, develop and be ready for the industry when they graduate. Unlike students studying in the university during academic semesters, students at internships function as both students and employees. There are certain considerations that we should bear in mind as we are coaching students on internships.

Workplace internships offer great learning opportunities for students to develop a growth mindset. As discussed in this chapter, we observed that students with a growth mindset received better ratings from their work supervisors in problem-solving and decision-making at the end of their internship programme, demonstrating that they were more open to challenges and experimentation in their pursuit of mastery goals. It is therefore important for university supervisors to work with the students and workplace supervisors through coaching and mentoring when a student struggles instead of offering immediate or direct solutions. Students who perceive challenges as too difficult or incapable of solving an issue can be coached into understanding the power of "not yet", encouraging them that the challenge can help them grow and develop new capabilities to succeed.

While we advocate coaching by the academic supervisors, there are some "not-to-coach" areas which supervisors should be mindful of. These include issues where ethical concerns require intervention from the university rather than having the student work out the issue through coaching. Some examples may include workplace bullying, sexual harassment, work practices that endanger the student or illegal activities happening at the workplace. If the student is truly distressed by such issues, academic supervisors would be their lifeline to intervene. Otherwise, the workplace is a truly authentic place to learn and grow through coaching.

Coaching Questions

Goal Questions

- Suppose this is a successful internship, at the end of the programme, what skills would you like to develop?
- From your experience thus far, what would you like to improve on?
- What makes this an important skill for you to develop?

Reality Questions

- What previous experience would you consider useful for this situation?
- Who are the key stakeholders you work with?
- What are some positive experiences at the workplace you have had thus far?
- For the professional skill you want to work on, where are you now on a scale of 1 to 10, with 1 being poor and 10 being excellent?

Option Questions

- How can you make the internship a success where you are able to achieve your developmental goals?
- What or who else at work would help in this situation?
- What would your work supervisor say about this suggestion?

Way Forward Questions

- What are some concrete steps we can take to bring this forward?
- What can increase your confidence to take those steps at the workplace?
- How would you know if you are successful in moving towards your goals?

Discussion Starters

- As an academic supervisor, how can you support students to make the best of their learnings from university and their workplace internship?
- What are key skills you would like to see students develop in work-based learning, and why do you deem them important?
- Where are some coachable moments in work-based learning and how can you draw them out in your coaching conversations with students?
- What are some perspectives you need to appreciate and consider about the workplace when coaching your student towards his or her preferred future?

References

Atkinson, A., Watling, C. J., & Brand, P. L. P. (2021). Feedback and coaching. *European Journal of Pediatrics*, *181*(2), 441–446. https://doi.org/10.1007/s00431-021-04118-8

Bayerlein, L. (2020). The impact of prior work-experience on student learning outcomes in simulated internships. *Journal of University Teaching & Learning Practice*, *17*(4), 44–61. https://doi.org/10.53761/1.17.4.4

Cronin, L., Allen, J., Ellison, P., Marchant, D., Levy, A., & Harwood, C. (2019). Development and initial validation of the life skills ability scale for higher education students. *Studies in Higher Education*, *46*(6), 1011–1024. https://doi.org/10.1080/03075079.2019.1672641

Dweck, C. (2006). *Mindset: The new psychology of success*. Random House.

Dweck, C. S., & Leggett, E. L. (1988). A social-cognitive approach to motivation and personality. *Psychological Review*, *95*(2), 256–273. https://doi.org/10.1037/0033-295X.95.2.256

Feldmann, L. (2016). Considerations in the design of WBL settings to enhance students' employability: A synthesis of individual and contextual perspectives. *Higher Education, Skills and Work-Based Learning*, *6*(2), 131–145. https://doi.org/10.1108/heswbl-09-2014-0044

Goller, M., Harteis, C., Gijbels, D., & Donche, V. (2020). Engineering students' learning during internships: Exploring the explanatory power of the job demands-control-support model. *Journal of Engineering Education*, *109*(2), 307–324. https://doi.org/10.1002/jee.20308

Green, B. P., Graybeal, P., & Madison, R. L. (2010). An exploratory study of the effect of professional internships on students' perception of the importance of employment traits. *Journal of Education for Business*, *86*(2), 100–110. https://doi.org/10.1080/08832323.2010.480992

Krackov, S. K., Pohl, H. S., Peters, A. S., & Sargeant, J. M. (2017). Feedback, reflection and coaching: a new model. In J. A. Dent, R. M. Harden, & D. Hunt (Eds), *A practical guide for medical teachers* (5th ed., pp. 281–288). Elsevier.

Luk, L. Y. Y., & Chan, C. K. Y. (2021). Students' learning outcomes from engineering internship: A provisional framework. *Studies in Continuing Education*, *44*(3), 526–545. https://doi.org/10.1080/0158037x.2021.1917536

Luthans, F., & Peterson, S. J. (2003). 360-degree feedback with systematic coaching: Empirical analysis suggests a winning combination. *Human Resource Management*, *42*(3), 243–256. https://doi.org/10.1002/hrm.10083

Maaravi, Y., Heller, B., Hochman, G., & Kanat-Maymon, Y. (2020). Internship not hardship: What makes interns in startup companies satisfied? *The Journal of Experimental Education*, *44*(3), 257–276. https://doi.org/10.1177/1053825920966351

Molyn, J. (2020). The role and effectiveness of coaching in increasing self-efficacy and employability efforts of higher education students. *Proceedings of the MIT LINC 2019 Conference, 3,* 178–187. https://doi.org/10.29007/294n

Ng, J., Yeo, M.-F., & Foo, Y. L. (2020). The integrated work study programme at Singapore Institute of Technology: More than a traditional internship model. In S. M. Lim, Y. L. Foo, H. T. Loh, & X. Deng (Eds), *Applied learning in higher education: Perspective, pedagogy, and practice* (pp. 17–26). Informing Science Press.

Peters, S., Clarebout, G., Aertgeerts, B., Michels, N., Pype, P., Stammen, L., & Roex, A. (2019). Provoking a conversation around students' and supervisors' expectations regarding workplace learning. *Teaching and Learning in Medicine, 32*(3), 282–293. https://doi.org/10.1080/10401334.2019.1704764

Sargeant, J. M., Mann, K. V., van der Vleuten, C. P., & Metsemakers, J. F. (2008). Reflection: A link between receiving and using assessment feedback. *Advances in Health Sciences Education, 14*(3), 399–410. https://doi.org/10.1007/s10459-008-9124-4

Schroth, H. (2019). Are you ready for Gen Z in the workplace? *California Management Review, 61*(3), 5–18. https://doi.org/10.1177/0008125619841006

Singapore Institute of Technology (n.d.). *Aircraft systems engineering: Developed in collaboration with SIA Engineering Company (SIAEC).* Retrieved December 26, 2023, from www.singaporetech.edu.sg/undergraduate-programmes/aircraft-systems-engineering

Tee, D., Barr, M., & van Nieuwerburgh, C. (2019). The experiences of educational coaches prior to their first placement: An interpretative phenomenological analysis. *International Journal of Evidence Based Coaching and Mentoring, 17*(2), 52–63. https://doi.org/10.24384/ssyk-hx16

Tudor, T. R. (2018). Fully integrating academic advising with career coaching to increase student retention, graduation rates and future job satisfaction: An industry approach. *Industry and Higher Education, 32*(2), 73–79. https://doi.org/10.1177/0950422218759928

Whitmore, J. (2017). *Coaching for performance: Growing human potential and purpose – The principles and practice of coaching and leadership* (4th ed.). CreateSpace Independent Publishing Platform.

World Economic Forum. (2023, May). *The future of jobs report 2023: Insight report.* www.weforum.org/reports/the-future-of-jobs-report-2023/in-full

10 Coaching in Clinical Supervision

Karina Dancza and Valerie P. C. Lim

Chapter Objectives

- To introduce the Professional Learning through Useful Support (PLUS) Framework to support clinical supervisors to enhance their supervisory sessions during clinical placements.
- To provide examples of how coaching and solution-focused approaches can be combined with critical supervisory focal points to support students' learning and professional development.
- To offer practical guidance on how universities can support clinical educators to use the PLUS Framework alongside coaching and solution-focused approaches to enhance their students' learning during clinical placements.

Keywords

clinical education
clinical supervision
coaching
feedback
solution-focused approach
supervisor guidance
reflection

Introduction

In this chapter, we will draw from our experience as clinicians and clinical supervisors and from our collective experiences as university educators in Occupational Therapy (Karina) and Speech and Language Therapy (Valerie) to describe how we support our students using coaching and solution-focused approaches during their clinical placements. We use the Professional Learning through Useful Support (PLUS) Framework (Dancza et al., 2021) to outline

DOI: 10.4324/9781003332176-13

practical guidance on how coaching and solution-focused approaches can be combined with our understanding of critical supervisory focal points to enhance student learning and professional development.

This chapter is intended as an introduction to coaching and student clinical supervision. To illustrate some key concepts, we reference a few frequently encountered scenarios in our supervisory practice. We appreciate that the supervisory context during clinical placements can be more varied and complex than the scenarios presented in this chapter. Nonetheless, we hope our scenarios present a helpful starting point for your consideration and reflection. We will begin this chapter by providing a brief overview of our professions, outlining what we mean by clinical education and clinical supervision, and introducing the Professional Learning through Useful Support (PLUS) Framework to structure supervision with students.

Occupational Therapy and Speech and Language Therapy

As health professional educators based in Singapore, we teach and prepare students for eventual registration as Allied Health Professionals so that they can enter the workforce as Occupational Therapists and Speech and Language Therapists.

A significant part of the education of Occupational Therapists and Speech and Language Therapists involves working alongside qualified health professionals in various settings, where students can apply their university learning to real-life situations (Health Education England, 2020). These experiences are called clinical education or placements.

Clinical Education

Clinical education for healthcare professionals (e.g. medical students, nursing students and allied health students) differs from regular university internships in several ways, particularly regarding safety and registration for practice. In clinical education, safety is a top priority. Students may have direct patient care responsibilities and, therefore, must be equipped with the necessary knowledge and skills to prevent harm to themselves, their colleagues and the people accessing their healthcare services. Students completing clinical education are also generally unpaid and closely supervised by qualified healthcare professionals who oversee the students' clinical activities (Gibson et al., 2018; Rodger et al., 2011).

Clinical education is also mandated before students graduate and register in their chosen profession. This registration ensures that students have met the required educational and national standards and have demonstrated the necessary skills to practice safely. Before graduation, students typically experience at least 800–1000 hours of work experience in various areas, such as hospitals, children's clinics or aged care facilities. Students are typically supervised by a qualified and experienced Occupational Therapist or Speech and Language Therapist based in the placement setting (Health Education England, 2020; Speech Pathology Australia, 2018; World Federation of Occupational Therapists, 2016).

Our role as university educators is to prepare students for clinical place-ments and help them apply their university learning in practice. We also guide the practising clinical supervisors in coaching and supporting students during their clinical education (Bivall et al., 2020). To do this, we use supervisory frameworks like the Professional Learning through Useful Support (PLUS) Framework (Dancza et al., 2021), which we will outline next.

Clinical Supervision and the Professional Learning through Useful Support (PLUS) Framework

Clinical supervision is a formal process of learning and professional develop-ment, and in the context of health professionals, is intended to promote opti-mal outcomes, safety and wellbeing of people who access services (Martin et al., 2021). Clinical supervision of students is often an extra role that

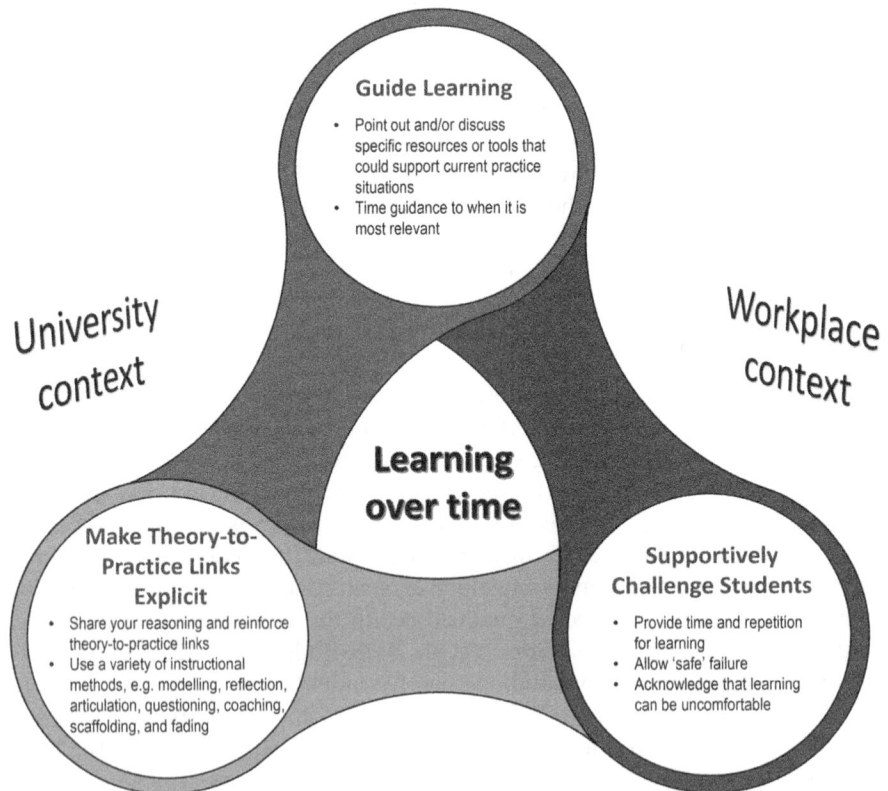

Figure 10.1 The Professional Learning through Useful Support (PLUS) Framework

Note: Used with permission of John Wiley & Sons Books, from Clinical Teacher Figure 2: The Professional Learning through Useful Support [PLUS] Framework. From "PLUS framework: Guidance for practice educators," by K. Dancza, J. Copley and M. Moran, 2021, *Clinical Teacher*, *18*(4), p. 6 (https://doi.org/10.1111/tct.13393). Permission conveyed through Copyright Clearance Center, Inc.

Occupational Therapists or Speech and Language Therapists take on in addition to their already busy roles in their respective healthcare, community and educational settings. The time spent in supervision is precious; hence, this time needs to be efficient and effective. Guidance is needed to support clinical supervisors in allocating their time and resources to areas more likely to promote student learning.

The Professional Learning through Useful Support (PLUS) Framework (Dancza et al., 2021) is one such support that I (Karina) developed within Occupational Therapy as part of my PhD research (Figure 10.1). The PLUS Framework highlights three focal points for clinical supervisors to enhance students' learning opportunities: (1) Guide Learning, (2) Make Theory-to-Practice Links Explicit, and (3) Supportively Challenge Students.

To help illustrate how the PLUS Framework can guide clinical supervision, we would like to introduce you to Riza, a health professional student on placement, and Sue, her clinical supervisor. We share the start of the story in Box 10.1.

In the following sections, we share how coaching and solution-focused approaches can be applied at each of the three focal points of the PLUS Framework. We continue to explore Riza and Sue's story to illustrate how this might look in practice. We start with Guide Learning.

Box 10.1 Introducing Riza and Sue

Riza is a healthcare professional student on clinical placement in an adult ward at Sunshine Hospital. It is early in week two of her clinical placement. Riza has observed her supervisor and conducted two patient assessments. So far, she has been doing relatively well for routine cases and has shown the ability to extract the relevant past medical and therapy history from the case notes, identify some knowledge gaps and ask relevant questions to fill in those gaps and provide a reasonable idea of what might be causing the patient's challenges. The next stage is for Riza to plan what to do in therapy, starting by setting some therapy targets related to a patient's goals, considering the context of the patient and any assessment information gathered.

After assessing Madam Low, an outpatient, Riza initially attempts to set therapy targets. Riza learns from Madam Low that she wants to go out with her friends and not stay at home all the time. Riza writes a therapy plan that involves Madam Low doing a range of daily exercises and gives it to Sue, her clinical supervisor, for feedback.

Sue reviews the plan and has concerns over Riza's therapy recommendations. They do not appear based on what Madam Low wanted to achieve in therapy, nor were they relevant to Madam Low's interests, diagnosis or home situation. Sue decides to use the **PLUS Framework** with coaching and solution-focused approaches to support Riza's progress in her placement.

Guide Learning

The primary role of a clinical supervisor is to guide students' learning. During clinical placements, students are novices in the setting and must fit into the working practices and apply their university-gained knowledge to their work. Clinical supervisors are critical in helping students make connections between the ideas they have been taught at university (out of a real-life context) and what they need to do in the workplace (in the real-life context) (Dunst et al., 2019; Gibson et al., 2018). However, educational theory suggests that applying knowledge from one context, such as in a university, into another context, such as a workplace, is complicated, uncommon and unpredictable (Evans & Guile, 2012).

The guidance provided by clinical supervisors needs to be timely and specific. Advice for students is more helpful when timed at a point where they can almost immediately apply it. Providing something specific, such as an article, book chapter, website, policy or technical paper, gives students a concrete place to start their investigations in an increasingly information-overloaded world. For example, clinical supervisors might share a specific technique for how to get to know a person accessing their services and establish a therapeutic relationship in the first week of the clinical placement (timely and specific guidance). The clinical supervisor can then build on this guidance as the student has had time to consolidate and practice the technique, reflecting an intentional and gradual release of information (Evans & Guile, 2012).

In Box 10.2, we share a conversation between Sue and Riza where Sue uses coaching and solution-focused principles to guide Riza's learning in planning therapy with Madam Low.

Box 10.2   How Sue Uses Coaching and Solution-Focused Principles to Guide Learning

Riza: Good morning, Ms Sue.

Sue: Good morning, Riza. I read your therapy recommendations for Madam Low and wanted to give you some feedback … You were specific and made a good start, so I understood what you planned to do. Please tell me more about how you decided on your therapy targets for Madam Low.

Riza: Well, Madam Low has had a stroke, and I know from the literature that she needs to do the therapy exercise with some intensity. So, I followed the standard exercise protocol (e.g. ten repetitions three times a day).

Sue: I see. In the last session, Madam Low's daughter was with her. Can you remember what her daughter mentioned about how things have been at home since her discharge?

Riza: Oh … she was not so motivated to do any exercise.

Sue: Yes. In my experience, there is usually a reason or a connection between motivation and therapy. I typically find out more about the patient and tailor my plans to suit their situation … Perhaps think of a time when you were motivated to do something or complete a task; what helped you to do it?

Riza: Oh … It was better when I found the task interesting or could see why it helped me do what I wanted.

Sue: Hmm… OK. What else?

Riza: (*pauses and thinks, Sue waits*) Erm … It was something I thought I could actually do, not too difficult or overwhelming.

Sue: OK. If you look again at your plans for Madam Low, is there anything you notice?

Riza: I guess it is only about the exercises, but I didn't think about Madam Low as a person, with other things going on besides her stroke.

Sue: That is a valuable insight. What frameworks or models have you been taught so far that help you to think about Madam Low more holistically?

Riza: Oh … I can't really think of anything right now … Is there something you use?

Sue: Do you recall a module you studied on Understanding Health? Was there anything introduced to you?

Riza: Yes! Now I recall, there are a few, but the one I can think of now is the ICF, International Classification of Functioning, Disability and Health framework. Yes, that might help. Can I have some time to review it and get back to you?

Sue: Sure, let's pick this up again on Thursday.

The conversation between Sue and Riza demonstrated a common scenario where Riza missed something vital in her practice when she did not consider Madam Low's motivation to do exercises in her therapy plan. Rather than pointing out the error directly, Sue asked coaching questions to draw Riza's attention to what she missed (*Can you remember what her daughter mentioned about how things have been at home since her discharge?*).

Sue went on to help Riza connect Madam Low's motivation with something that Riza may have experienced herself. This helped Riza to understand the patient's perspective (theory-of-mind), to appreciate how Madam Low may be feeling and to facilitate thinking about exceptions or things that could be done differently (*Think of a time when you were motivated to do or complete a task, what helped you to do it?*).

In addition, Sue also guided Riza to think about a specific idea from her university learning that could help her think through this workplace scenario (*What frameworks or models have you been taught so far that help you to think about Madam Low more holistically?*). Riza could not think of anything immediately until Sue asked what she had learnt in a specific module (*Do you recall a module you studied on Understanding Health?*). Once Riza was guided towards a particular idea, she recalled the International Classification of Functioning, Disability and Health (ICF) framework. She started to think about its connection with this current situation.

Through this guidance and a re-focus on previous personal success/exceptions, Riza could conclude what she missed (*It is only about the exercises*). Importantly, as she came up with this herself (solution-focused), she will likely remember it the next time she works with a patient.

As Sue guided Riza to think about the ICF Framework, she moved on to our next focal point: **Make Theory-to-Practice Links Explicit**. We will further explore how she guides Riza to link a theory she has been introduced to at university with what she needs to do in practice in the next section, then return to Sue and Riza for their next supervision conversation.

Make Theory-to-Practice Links Explicit

As a more experienced person in the profession and the setting, clinical supervisors can quickly decide what to do. They incorporate a range of information, such as knowledge of theories, therapeutic techniques, diagnostic criteria, previous experiences, information from the person accessing services and many other sources (Parnell et al., 2019; Smyth & McCabe, 2017).

Knowing what information the supervisor has drawn on to make specific decisions is challenging for a student. Indeed, many experienced supervisors may not be consciously aware of all the elements they have considered when making each decision (Richmond et al., 2020). Making this implicit decision-making process more explicit helps students make their own connections and understand how their university learning informs their workplace practice (Dancza et al., 2019).

To support students in connecting theory with practice, clinical supervisors may need to review any significant theories or concepts the students are familiar with and have conversations with students about how knowing that information informed the decisions that were made (Warren et al., 2016). For example, clinical supervisors could explain to a student which theory they used to inform their choice of assessment tool. They could also use a framework to demonstrate how it helped them to make sense of the findings from the assessment and inform what could be done next. These supervision discussions reflect transformative learning theory, where supervisors engage students in ongoing two-way dialogue, encouraging new ideas and learning (Meyer & Timmermans, 2016).

We return to the next supervision conversation between Riza and Sue in Box 10.3, where Sue illustrates how she uses coaching and solution-focused approaches with Riza to continue to help her make theory-to-practice links explicit.

Box 10.3   How Sue Uses Coaching and Solution-Focused Principles to Make Theory-To-Practice Links Explicit

Sue: Nice to see you again, Riza. How did you go with your research about the International Classification of Functioning, Disability and Health or ICF framework and Madam Low's therapy plan?

Riza: Hello, Ms Sue. Well, I guess I did OK. I found the notes I had and searched online for ICF and stroke. I couldn't find anything that matched Madam Low's situation and an appropriate therapy plan, though …

Sue: I have a good article about the ICF framework and therapy planning that has helped others. Would you like me to share it with you?

Riza: Yes, please! That would be great.

Sue: You know, sometimes we do get stuck. In the past, what worked for you to become unstuck?

Riza: Hmm … I remember being stuck during my previous placement when I tried to build rapport with a caregiver, which didn't go too well. I discussed what happened with my friend and tried to read up more independently.

Sue: And how did that work out for you?

Riza: OK … but I still didn't really know what to do.

Sue: Was there anyone else you could talk to about this?

Riza: Maybe I should have asked my clinical supervisor at the time …

Sue: It is OK to say, "I'm stuck. Can you point me in the right direction? Or do you have something I can read about developing rapport with caregivers?"

Riza: Yes, yes. OK (smiling). Thank you. … Hmmm … would you mind sharing your use of the ICF with one of your patients? I think it would help me to see how you frame a patient using this framework.

Sue: Yes, sure. Let's get the article, and I can tell you about Mr Tan, the person you sat in on the initial assessment with me the other day … [Sue and Riza continued the conversation, with Sue talking through each element of the ICF and providing examples of what she did and how she was making decisions about the therapy plan for Mr Tan.]

Riza: Thank you! That was really insightful. I think I will be able to prepare something similar for Madam Low. Can I bring this back to you in our next session?

Sue: Yes, no problem.

Box 10.3 illustrates how Sue provided coaching to Riza by inquiring about her current understanding of the ICF framework, which Riza had researched. Sue then proceeded to enhance Riza's comprehension and application of the framework while offering techniques for seeking assistance.

Sue provided an open platform where teaching (rather than testing the student) could occur. (*I have a good article about the ICF framework and therapy planning that has helped others. Would you like me to share it with you?*) She gave a few ideas to Riza about what she could do when she feels stuck (*It is fine to say, "I'm a bit stuck, can you point me in the right direction? Or do you have something I can read about developing rapport with caregivers?"*), Moreover, this opened the door for Riza to ask Sue about her expert professional reasoning and how she uses the ICF framework to help her therapy plans. Sue then coached Riza by making her theory-to-practice links explicit to Riza using the example of Mr Tan. Riza could then apply her new insight to develop her plans with Madam Low.

In our final focal point of the PLUS Framework, we see how Sue supportively challenges Riza to put her plans into action so that she can learn from her own experience how effective they are.

Supportively Challenge Students

The final focus point in the PLUS Framework concentrates on how clinical supervisors supportively challenge students to enhance their learning. This supportive challenge includes giving students the space and time to try their ideas and learn from their successes and mistakes in a controlled situation.

Allowing students to follow through with a plan when a clinical supervisor can see potential issues can be uncomfortable for the clinical supervisor. It may be more intuitive to correct the students' plan or take over a session if the student appears to be struggling so that there is more likelihood of success. However, by preventing *any* issues from happening or acting as a safety net by taking over a session, the student may not feel the responsibility of the situation or be aware of the consequences of their actions until the student is in a more independent and potentially riskier situation when the supervisor is no longer present. Significant learning is possible when students can try their ideas, see what happens, and adjust in the moment if needed (Henriksen et al., 2021; Manalo & Kapur, 2018). There are, of course, safety and ethical limits to this approach. However, selecting low-stakes situations and doing an appropriate risk assessment, allowing students to test their thinking and reasoning in practice can enhance their overall abilities as developing healthcare professionals (Klasen & Lingard, 2019).

Clinical supervisors also recognise that students need considerable time to repeatedly practice skills (repetition of concepts) for deep learning. This is particularly noticeable when students must think for themselves rather than follow established routines (Dancza et al., 2019). This supportive learning space is achieved through supervisors offering emotional support and challenging students to analyse, reflect and make their own decisions about their practice. This resonates with threshold concepts literature, where learning is viewed as an embodied and sometimes uncomfortable experience rather than only an intellectual or cognitive process (Meyer & Timmermans, 2016).

Recognising that deep learning can be an emotional and tiring experience helps clinical supervisors create an optimal balance between the productivity of students working with people accessing the service and thinking time. Talking about how learning can be uncomfortable at times is also a helpful approach, and this can reassure students that it is a typical experience when engaging in deep learning (Gribble et al., 2016). Clinical supervisors are also encouraged to seek support, acknowledging the emotional load associated with supporting students' learning (Morgan et al., 2018; Warren et al., 2016). Box 10.4 illustrates how Sue supportively challenged Riza in the next instalment of our story.

In Box 10.4, Sue uses coaching and solution-focused strategies to supportively challenge Riza to talk with Madam Low about her therapy plans. We can tell that Riza feels out of her comfort zone. Still, Sue has evaluated the situation and determined that having a conversation with Riza is low risk for Madam Low and that Riza needs to gain experience in explaining her therapy plans and involving Madam Low in the decision-making process. Sue has also supported Riza in evolving her plans to an acceptable standard before sharing them with Madam Low (the timeframes and activities are more reasonable than her initial therapy plans).

Box 10.4   How Sue Uses Coaching and Solution-Focused Principles to Supportively Challenge Riza

Sue: Hello Riza! Thanks for sharing your updated therapy plan for Madam Low. This is looking much better – well done. I notice that you have used the ICF framework and considered Madam Low's situation more, like going out with her friends to the coffee shop after a morning walk.

Riza: Yes, your article and our previous discussion was very useful. Thanks.

Sue: Can I ask you about the timeframes you have suggested here? Considering the number of sessions she might have with you in the next three weeks, how do you plan this out from session to session? I will give you some time to write the plan, and I will return in 10 minutes.

[After checking the patient appointments, Riza spends 10 minutes working out the session plans and realises that Madam Low only has four sessions in the next three weeks. When she writes out the session targets, she also realises Madam Low will only be ready to go out independently after the end of four sessions. Sue re-enters the room.]

Riza: I can now see that four sessions will not be enough for Madam Low to achieve her goal. I didn't consider how many sessions she had and what she could do within that time. That was a mistake, and I feel bad I didn't see it earlier.

Sue: It is all part of the learning to have a go, and now you can review what you need to do next. It's hard to remember everything, but hopefully, this is something you can look out for in the future … What do you think you want to do next?

Riza: I would like to update the plan to make it more realistic. Then I would like to check it again with you. Is that OK?

Sue: Yes, sure. But I also think you will need to check your plan with someone else … (*Riza looks puzzled*) … who is most impacted by the therapy plans?

Riza: Hmmm … Madam Low, I guess?

Sue: Yes, would you like to talk with her and see what she thinks?

Riza: (*Riza looks nervous*) … I think she should be involved, but I am not very confident I would know what to say …

Sue: That's OK. You are still learning, so it won't always come so quickly and naturally. How might you prepare for this conversation?

Riza: I could write some questions and prepare something I could share with Madam Low.

Sue: A good start. What would you like to see happen regarding your communication of the therapy plans with Madam Low by the end of this week?

Riza: I want to be clear about what I am suggesting and why I am suggesting it when I speak with Madam Low. I also want to listen to Madam Low's views to plan a way forward together. Sometimes, I get caught up thinking about what I am saying because I don't always pay enough attention to what a patient is telling me.

Sue: That is really insightful, Riza. That will help you know where to focus your learning. So, what difference would it make for you … if you were to achieve this?

Riza: I will feel better … more confident … that I am getting this.

Sue: I like that determination, Riza. What usually helps you to get a hang of things faster?

Riza: I like to practise … and practise.

Sue: OK, so what are your plans to practise?

Riza: Maybe I can role-play with my classmates, going through things together to make sure I'm on the right track … maybe I can discuss cases with Peter (another student at the same placement) since he will have had similar experiences. Then maybe I can have a practice with you … before I speak with Madam Low?

Sue: Sounds like a plan. Let's do this practice tomorrow and then you can speak with Madam Low the day after.

Riza: OK (*laughs a bit nervously*).

Sue tells Riza that she knows she may feel challenged in this situation and that this type of deep learning can be uncomfortable. Solution-focused questions (*What would you like to see happen at the end of the week? What difference would it make? What helps you?*) helped Riza with goal setting and envisioning how she would feel once she achieves her goal. It also allowed Riza to state what learning methods helped her succeed in the past.

Sue also enabled Riza to have the time for repetition of learning before her conversation with Madam Low with her classmate and herself. Sue also knows that Riza can practise this type of conversation with other patients while on placement, so Riza can learn from each interaction and consolidate her skills using practice, reflection and feedback opportunities. In the final conversation between Riza and Sue, we join them for a feedback session after Riza's conversation with Madam Low (Box 10.5).

Box 10.5   How Sue Uses Coaching and Solution-Focused Principles in a Feedback Session

Sue: How did it go with Madam Low?

Riza: I think it went pretty well. I was really nervous, but once I started sharing my plans, I could see that she was really excited about getting back to do the things that were important to her. That made me feel like I was on the right track.

Sue: That sounds really positive. What about when you listened to Madam Low's views? How did that go?

Riza: Well, that was OK, but not great. I think I was so excited to share, and Madam Low was really nice about my plans, that I may not have given her the space to share her views fully.

Sue: That sounds like something to think more about then? What might you do differently next time?

Riza: Well, maybe I should have paused a bit more during the conversation and asked Madam Low what she thought? From our last conversation, I really wanted to ensure that it would be meaningful for her. I think I need to think about this a bit more, and maybe read up on that motivational interviewing technique you shared at the team meeting yesterday …

Sue: I like that idea. So, to recap, what is one or two main things you will take away from this experience?

Riza: I think the main learning for me is that I need to think about people as more than just their diagnosis, and to involve them in the planning of any therapy sessions, as it shouldn't just be my plans driving therapy. But to do this properly, I want to work more on my conversational skills and how I can create the space for joint decision-making with my patients.

Sue: Thank you for sharing, and I look forward to our next chat.

You may have noticed that in the feedback conversation in Box 10.5, Sue did not need to offer Riza advice. Riza was familiar with the coaching approach and was able to come up with her own ideas and plans for what she learnt and what she would do next. Some well-chosen questions from Sue facilitated Riza's reflections, and Sue did not see the need to add further. Sue also planned for Riza to have more opportunities to practice her skills throughout the placement.

As we have demonstrated with Sue and Risa, the PLUS Framework's focal points and the subsequent strategies associated with each point offer clinical educators a structure and flexibility to adapt what is required for each student's learning, considering the influence of the university and workplace contexts. The PLUS Framework is one way to support students and supervisors during placement learning and coaching, and solution-focused approaches complement how this is used in practice. Clinical supervision is, however, a complex activity to do well. Therefore, it is important that clinical supervisors continue to enhance their supervisory skills and expertise, but to do this, they also require support (Dancza et al., 2022). This can be achieved through discussions with supervisors, peers, and a community of practice. Box 10.6 offers a few questions that may help get coaching conversations going using the PLUS Framework.

Box 10.6   Coaching Questions incorporating the PLUS Framework

Guide Learning

- What do you think were the key elements of this situation?
- Think of a time where you have learnt or experienced something about these elements. What helped?
- How might that knowledge help you? (If needed, you may need to help the student identify what was important in the situation, such as communication skills, following a process, applying a theory, etc. and how these elements connect with their present situation.)

Make Theory-to-Practice Links Explicit

- Can you recall any theoretical frameworks or models you've learned that could help in this situation? (If needed, you can orientate the student to a particular topic, theory or subject they have learnt.)

Supportively Challenge Students

- What knowledge, skills or mindset would you like to develop during this experience?
- What would you notice if you were making process towards these goals?
- What can you or we do differently to help you develop and remember this knowledge, skill or mindset?
- What opportunities can we create to help you to try out and practise this new knowledge, skill or mindset?

Conclusion

This chapter introduced the Professional Learning through Useful Support (PLUS) Framework to enhance student learning and professional development during clinical placements. Using a case scenario of a student, Riza, we described how coaching and solution-focused approaches can be combined with critical supervisory focal points to support students in their clinical practice. We then offered practical guidance on how university educators can support clinical supervisors to use coaching and solution-focused approaches with their students during clinical placements.

Becoming flexible with the PLUS Framework and solution-focused approaches to coaching and how to transition between the two in real-life clinical supervisory practice is a supervisory skill which we know will improve with more practice and experience. While the PLUS Framework has been developed within a health context, its flexibility may offer potential structure when used alongside coaching and solution-focused approaches in professions beyond health.

Discussion Starters

Here are some suggested conversation starters and coaching questions to help clinical supervisors reflect on their practice, identify areas for growth and development, and incorporate the PLUS Framework into their supervisory practice.

- What do you think are the most important qualities of an effective clinical supervisor?
- What are some strategies you use to help students reflect on their practice?
- How can you apply the PLUS Framework, coaching and solution-focused questions in your future supervisory interactions and feedback?

References

Bivall, A.-C., Gustavsson, M., & Lindh Falk, A. (2020). Conditions for collaboration between higher education and healthcare providers organising clinical placements. *Higher Education, Skills and Work-Based Learning, 11*(4), 798–810. https://doi.org/10.1108/HESWBL-09-2020-0201

Dancza, K., Copley, J., & Moran, M. (2019). Occupational therapy student learning on role-emerging placements in schools. *British Journal of Occupational Therapy, 82*(9), 567–577. https://doi.org/10.1177/0308022619840167

Dancza, K., Copley, J., & Moran, M. (2021). PLUS framework: Guidance for practice educators. *The Clinical Teacher, 18*(4), 431–438. https://doi.org/10.1111/tct.13393

Dancza, K., Tempest, S., Volkert, A., Baird, J. M., Taylor, G. M., O'Dea, Á., Harvey, S., Kramer-Roy, D., & Hirani, N. J. (2022). An introduction to the 3Cs for effective supervision. In K. Dancza, A. Volkert, & S. Tempest (Eds), *Supervision for occupational therapy: Practical guidance for supervisors and supervisees* (pp. 48–63). Routledge. https://doi.org/10.4324/9781003092544-3

Dunst, C. J., Hamby, D. W., Howse, R. B., Wilkie, H., & Annas, K. (2019). Research synthesis of meta-analyses of preservice teacher preparation practices in higher education. *Higher Education Studies*, *10*(1), 29–47. https://doi.org/10.5539/hes.v10n1p29

Evans, K., & Guile, D. (2012). Putting different forms of knowledge to work in practice. In J. Higgs, R. Barnett, S. Billett, M. Hutchings, & F. Trede (Eds), *Practice-based education: Perspectives and strategies* (pp. 113–130). Sense Publishers. https://doi.org/10.1007/978-94-6209-128-3_9

Gibson, S. J., Porter, J., Anderson, A., Bryce, A., Dart, J., Kellow, N., Meiklejohn, S., Volders, E., Young, A., & Palermo, C. (2018). Clinical educators' skills and qualities in allied health: A systematic review. *Medical Education in Review*, *53*(5), 432–442. https://doi.org/10.1111/medu.13782

Gribble, N., Ladyshewsky, R. K., & Parsons, R. (2016). Fluctuations in the emotional intelligence of therapy students during clinical placements: Implication for educators, supervisors, and students. *Journal of Interprofessional Care*, *31*(1), 8–17. https://doi.org/10.1080/13561820.2016.1244175

Health Education England. (2020, August). *Current placement expectations of AHP regulators and professional bodies.* www.hee.nhs.uk/our-work/allied-health-professions/helping-ensure-essential-supply-ahps/placement-expansion-innovation/current-placement-expectations-ahp-regulators

Henriksen, D., Henderson, M., Creely, E., Carvalho, A. A., Cernochova, M., Dash, D., Davis, T., & Mishra, P. (2021). Creativity and risk-taking in teaching and learning settings: Insights from six international narratives. *International Journal of Educational Research Open*, *2*, 100024. https://doi.org/10.1016/j.ijedro.2020.100024

Klasen, J. M., & Lingard, L. A. (2019). Allowing failure for educational purposes in postgraduate clinical training: A narrative review. *Medical Teacher*, *41*(11), 1263–1269. https://doi.org/10.1080/0142159X.2019.1630728

Manalo, E., & Kapur, M. (2018). The role of failure in promoting thinking skills and creativity: New findings and insights about how failure can be beneficial for learning. *Thinking Skills and Creativity*, *30*, 1–6. https://doi.org/10.1016/j.tsc.2018.06.001

Martin, P., Lizarondo, L., Kumar, S., & Snowdon, D. (2021). Impact of clinical supervision on healthcare organisational outcomes: A mixed methods systematic review. *PLoS One*, *16*(11), e0260156. https://doi.org/10.1371/journal.pone.0260156

Meyer, J. H. F., & Timmermans, J. A. (2016). Integrated threshold concept knowledge. In R. Land, J. H. F. Meyer, & M. T. Flanagan (Eds), *Threshold concepts in practice* (pp. 25–38). Sense Publishers. https://doi.org/10.1007/978-94-6300-512-8_3

Morgan, K., Reidlinger, D. P., Sargeant, S., Crane, L., & Campbell, K. L. (2018). Challenges in preparing the dietetics workforce of the future: An exploration of dietetics educators' experiences. *Nutrition & Dietetics*, *76*(4), 382–391. https://doi.org/10.1111/1747-0080.12438

Parnell, T., Whiteford, G., & Wilding, C. (2019). Differentiating occupational decision-making and occupational choice. *Journal of Occupational Science*, *26*(3), 442–448. https://doi.org/10.1080/14427591.2019.1611472

Richmond, A., Cooper, N., Gay, S., Atiomo, W., & Patel, R. (2020). The student is key: A realist review of educational interventions to develop analytical and non-analytical clinical reasoning ability. *Medical Education*, *54*(8), 709–719. https://doi.org/10.1111/medu.14137

Rodger, S., Fitzgerald, C., Davila, W., Millar, F., & Allison, H. (2011). What makes a quality occupational therapy practice placement? Students' and practice educators' perspectives. *Australian Occupational Therapy Journal*, *58*(3), 195–202. https://doi.org/10.1111/j.1440-1630.2010.00903.x

Smyth, O., & McCabe, C. (2017). Think and think again! Clinical decision making by advanced nurse practitioners in the emergency department. *International Emergency Nursing*, *31*, 72–74. https://doi.org/10.1016/j.ienj.2016.08.001

Speech Pathology Australia. (2018, August). *Clinical education in Australia: Building a profession for the future.* https://speechpathologyaustralia.cld.bz/Speak-Out-August-2018/22/

Warren, A., Dancza, K., McKay, E., Taylor, A., Moran, M., Copley, J., & Rodger, S. (2016). Supervising role emerging placements: A CPD opportunity that supports innovation in practice. *World Federation of Occupational Therapists Bulletin, 72*(1), 35–37. https://doi.org/10.1080/14473828.2016.1160992

World Federation of Occupational Therapists. (2016, March). *Minimum standards for education of occupational therapists.* https://wfot.org/resources/new-minimum-standards-for-the-education-of-occupational-therapists-2016-e-copy

11 Career Coaching and the Application of Career Theories in Higher Education

Boon Yong Kwok, Jeffrey Guan Ching Thng, Gin Yong Ong and Weili Zhang

---

Chapter Objectives

- To identify the infusion of career development theories in the design of career education and career coaching.
- To examine the application of career development theories in practice.
- To discuss the importance of theory-informed career coaching practice in higher education.

Keywords
career coaching
career development theories
career education
coach–client relationship
happenstance
higher education
internship
transition

Introduction

This chapter looks at how career development theories are useful in designing and enacting career education curriculum and career coaching services offered to students in their undergraduate years in university. In the discussion of career development, we extend the boundaries beyond work readiness upon graduation to include students' pre-graduation internship opportunities and their career journey after joining the workforce. The career development consultation with a career coach is a theory-informed practice, and it involves a discovery of the student's interests and values, in addition to skills remediation and gap identification for the chosen path. In particular, the influence career coaches have over the students is significant and cannot be understated. The career coach does not

DOI: 10.4324/9781003332176-14

only open the doors to the industry, but also the doors to self-realisation especially in times of doubt when external narratives go against their beliefs.

Career Coaching Process

It is important to look at career education for university students holistically, transcending beyond the university years, because the knowledge, skills and attitudes for career wayfinding that students acquire will continue to serve them when they transit to the workplace and beyond. Career coaches must help students in "embracing career resilience and not just job stability" (Forward Singapore Workgroup, 2023).

Managing career coaching cases in a university can be similar with respect to the processes involved, and yet each one is very different due to the diverse population of students and their individual contexts. While there is no one-size-fits-all kind of coaching, we recommend four fundamental steps in the career coaches' coaching process: connection, clarification, facilitation and follow-through.

Connection

Connecting with the student is a critical step because if there is no connection, rapport cannot be built. Without rapport, there is no trust between the career coach and the student. Establishing a positive connection with the student empowers the career coach with a sense of purpose and a state of flow during the coaching process. The career coach will become more empathetic towards their student (Braun, 2022). A connection can be established through reflective listening. Reflective listening is a communication method that involves two steps: first, trying to understand what the student is saying, followed by summarising to ensure you got it right. It is a more specific way of listening when compared to general active listening (Kohli, 2016). With reflective listening comes genuine empathy, where the student feels they are truly being heard. Such sincerity from the career coach allows the student to open up and have more confidence in the coaching conversation.

Clarification

One of the greatest pitfalls in career coaching is not accurately identifying and addressing the student's real issue early, at the beginning of the coaching session. This results in the conversation going in different directions and may end up doing a disservice to the student, besides draining the career coach.

Cox (2013), and Conoley and Conoley (2009) identified four purposes of clarification in the coaching process, which can be applied to career coaching for students:

- To allow the student to feel acknowledged
- To resolve ambiguity and identify the actual issue

- To allow the student to undergo self-discovery through greater awareness and agreement on the actual issue
- To empower the student for an effective coaching process

Facilitation

Upon confirming the actual issue that the student wants to work on, the career coach helps them to identify actionable steps to take to address their issue. The GROW model, developed by Sir John Whitmore, is used widely by the coaching community to facilitate the coaching process (Kunos, 2017). Readers can refer to Chapter 2 of the book for more in-depth discussion. The four GROW steps are Goal, Reality, Options and Way-forward, and can be applied to career coaching:

- Goal – to define and clarify the objective of the career coaching session, where the career coach can ask questions, such as:
  - What career goals do you want to achieve in the short or long term?
  - How will you know if you have achieved your career goal?
  - What is in it for you when you attain your career goal?

- Reality – to explore the current situation and/or circumstances, where the career coach can ask:
  - What do you know about your present career situation?
  - What job search strategies have you tried so far?
  - What are some challenges you could face?

- Options – to gather alternative solutions and opportunities, where the career coach can ask:
  - What career or job search resources do you already have access to?
  - What other career or job search support do you need?
  - Who could be of help to offer guidance and support?

- Way-forward – to confirm how the client wants to move forward, where the coach can ask:
  - Which career option looks most viable at this point?
  - What is one thing you can do now to bring you one step closer to your career goal?
  - What is one thing you can do to overcome one or more of the challenges?

Follow-through

At this stage, the student should have developed an action plan based on what has been discussed (Hannum & Hoole, 2009). Without a clear action plan to follow through after the career coaching session, the student is more likely to lose momentum due to procrastination or doubt. Ideally, the career goal should be specific and measurable as it allows for a closer and targeted follow-up subsequently with regards to their progress and the process.

Career Readiness Curriculum and Example of Coaching Practice in a University

This section shares the approach that the career coaching team from Centre of Career Readiness (CCR) at Singapore Institute of Technology (SIT) takes for preparing students for their careers. Taking reference from the university's mission and applied learning pedagogy, the team identified critical milestones in the students' undergraduate journey to engage them purposefully from their first day as freshmen, through their work attachment, to their graduation (Ng et al., 2020). This is illustrated in Figure 11.1. The roadmap highlights the different touchpoints that are important in preparing students beyond the 1:1 experience of career coaching.

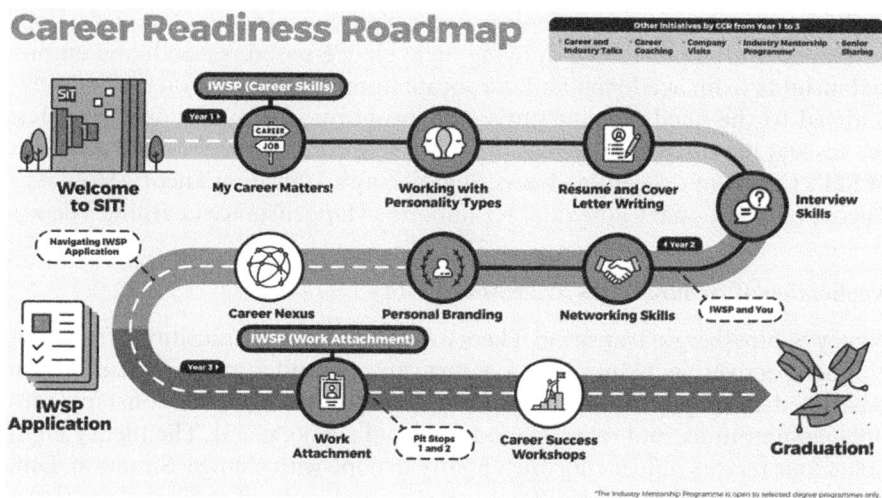

Figure 11.1 Singapore Institute of Technology's Career Readiness Roadmap

According to the Center for Credentialing & Education (2023), the touchpoints with students are important from a professional angle where career development support is made readily available throughout their journey, be they employability skills (résumé writing, interview skills, networking skills and personal branding) or profiling assessments (personality types). The importance of career planning and management is communicated and reinforced during student consultations with their career coaches. There are ample opportunities for students to apply their acquired skills at career networking events, including talks, fairs and industry mentorship programmes, in addition to their work attachment.

All students in SIT undergo work attachment, also known as Integrated Work Study Programme (IWSP), which is either 8 or 12 months in duration. Students are offered opportunities to connect with their career coaches, and to reflect and share on their work experience when they return to campus for "Pit Stops" during their work attachment (see Figure 11.1). More crucially, in the workshop towards the end of students' work attachment ("Pit Stop 2"), labour market information in the areas of relevant specialisations is shared. The career coach emphasises transition planning and prepares students to think about their career aspirations, creating an action plan for their transition from university to the workplace, especially if they have not already done so themselves.

Fundamental coaching skills, along with knowledge of the industry and organisational recruitment practices, a professional mindset, practical wisdom and positivity, make an effective university career coach. An understanding and application of career development theories will further empower the career coaches to confidently work with diverse cohorts of students and to adeptly deal with the plethora of cases they will encounter.

SIT's career readiness curriculum and career coaching practices have been developed and implemented drawing on evidence-based research and empirical insights from academia and corporate human resource practices contextualised to the needs of our university programmes and student profiles. We discuss the three key theories that have shaped the processes and practices of SIT's Centre of Career Readiness: Schlossberg's Transition Theory, Holland's Theory of Vocational Choice and Krumboltz's Happenstance Learning Theory.

Application of Schlossberg's Transition Theory

Nancy Schlossberg's Transition Theory (1984) examines transitions from several perspectives, including type, context, process and impact. Transition can be defined as "any event or non-event resulting in changed relationships, routines, assumptions, and roles" (Goodman et al., 2006, p. 33). The theory highlights four factors influencing one's ability to cope with change: Situation, Self, Support and Strategies. The different triggers and levels of resilience, resources and coping mechanisms available for employment by individuals can explain why different individuals react differently to the same transition, or why the same person may have a different response at another point in time.

We highlight one factor, Support, which is critical for students in the form of the available assistance and resources as part of university services (Evans et al., 1998). At SIT, the career coaching and employability skills workshops are available to the students at different stages of their transition from freshmen to co-workers; however, not all students may see the importance of these transitional support interventions immediately or they may not see how they are impacted by their actions (or inactions) in areas such as interview preparation and networking opportunities. Career coaches thus have a crucial role to play with just-in-time support, in preparing the students for their work attachment and beyond. Such ad-hoc consultations after career readiness workshops enable the coach and the student relationship to grow into one that is professionally respectful and beneficial, as the student progresses and matures over time on their career path.

A student may encounter a non-event transition, which is an occurrence that was expected but did not happen or was contrary to what was hoped for. Schlossberg (1984) is useful in helping students see that non-events can matter as much as the events that led to the state of transition in their life. Students are encouraged to see their career coaches to help them identify coping resources from their own self and their support, and for further recommendation of strategies. Students may be in a state of transition without knowing except for the emotions they may experience, for example, when they are struggling to secure their work attachment after submitting their résumés or going for interviews, or when they are released by their work attachment employers in situations not related to disciplinary issues. The career coach who knows Schlossberg's Transition Theory will be in a better position to support the student.

Application of Holland's Theory of Vocational Choice

John Holland's Theory of Vocational Choice (1997) often serves as a useful framework to help students check their career or degree programme fit when they are in doubt and to help them plan out the next actionable steps to take. His RIASEC profiling tool, which is based on the supposition that individuals are most satisfied and successful in work environments that match their personality types, is used in SIT and more widely by Singapore's public administration service (Government of Singapore, 2023).

Each of the six RIASEC codes corresponds to distinct characteristics and preferences:

- R: Realistic individuals are practical and hands-on
- I: Investigative individuals are analytical and curious
- A: Artistic individuals are creative and expressive
- S: Social individuals are compassionate and cooperative
- E: Enterprising individuals are assertive and persuasive
- C: Conventional individuals are detail oriented and organised

This tool comprises a self-reporting assessment that prompts students to reflect on their career interests, working preferences and work activities. By analysing their responses, students will gain insights into their vocational personality and undertake a more informed career exploration with the help of the career coach.

The RIASEC profiling tool can also serve as a foundation for career coaching conversations and comprehensive academic planning. The career coach can work with the student in aligning their current and near-future academic pursuits with their identified career interest to further enhance their immediate career readiness. They can then offer specific coursework or electives and take up relevant extracurricular activities in the short term. In Box 11.1, we illustrate with a case study where the RIASEC profiling tool provided the much-needed objective evidence that the student's career interests and work values are indeed aligned to her choice of degree programme.

Box 11.1 Coaching of a Struggling Student

This is a case of Lisa, a health science student who was struggling to cope with her schoolwork and the demands of clinical placement. She was initially sceptical about how career coaching could help to address her increasing conviction that the programme she was in was not the right course for her. Through a series of career coaching conversations, the career coach concluded that, in his professional judgement, the student's declining grades had led her to perceive that she had chosen the wrong degree programme, that she could not master the competencies needed to perform in her clinical placement, and as a result, Lisa lost interest in her studies. It was a negative self-perpetuating cycle.

The career coach employed Schlossberg's Transition Theory (1984) primarily at the initial stage of facilitation and identified the Self as the major factor among the four (the three others being Situation, Support and Strategies) in influencing Lisa's ability to cope with her reality revolving around schoolwork and clinical placement. During the subsequent sessions in the second half of facilitation, the career coach encouraged Lisa to explore her career interests and to understand her own strengths and work values using Holland's RIASEC profiling tool.

At the end of her coaching sessions, Lisa was reassured of her decision to embark on her chosen programme and was more optimistic about her clinical placement. The career coach was able to bring Lisa out of the negative self-perpetuating cycle by applying the theories and tools of Schlossberg (1984) and Holland (1997).

Application of Krumboltz's Happenstance Learning Theory (HLT)

Theories can help career coaches to make visible the undercurrents that could otherwise only be felt by students who are submerged in various states of negativity or uncertainty. We can see the career coach as a swim coach, metaphorically teaching the students not only to stay afloat and swim far, but also most importantly to first overcome the psychological barrier of dipping one's head underwater. A trained career coach should thus be well versed in career development theories which may comprise some elements of education psychology. One significant career development theory that draws on education psychology is John Krumboltz's Happenstance Learning Theory (HLT) (2008).

According to Krumboltz (2008), the complex interaction of planned and unplanned actions in response to self-initiated and circumstantial situations that can bring about unpredictable consequences can be labelled as happenstance. Krumboltz's HLT posits that we cannot always plan for things that will happen, which are results of what we do based on the decisions we make due to various factors such as genetic influences and the environment, but perhaps more importantly, what we have experienced or learnt before in school, situations or by observations. It is then important to plan for one's reaction to unplanned happenings, because "every situation can be seen as presenting potential opportunities if individuals can recognize them and then take action to capitalize on them" (Krumboltz, 2008, p. 136).

Krumboltz (2008) presents three steps in guiding one towards greater control of unplanned events:

1 Before any unplanned event:

   a One should take actions that position them to experience it. This means to be ready for unplanned event anytime, every time, and it is possible only if they possess the four key attitudes of curiosity, persistence, flexibility, and optimism (Jordan & Marinaccio, 2020).

   b During the event:

      i One should remain alert and sensitive to recognise potential opportunities.

   c After the event:

      i One should initiate actions that enable them to benefit from it.

According to Jordan and Marinaccio (2020), it is essential to foster the four key attitudes of curiosity, persistence, flexibility, and optimism for unexpected events. The question then is how students can cultivate these attitudes. Based on HLT, to identify and create career opportunities, five Happenstance skills are required. These five skills correspond with the four key attitudes, with the addition of "risk taking" (Mitchell et al., 1999). Career coaches can assist their students to develop and deploy the following five Happenstance skills in their job search and career development:

• Curiosity: exploring new learning opportunities
• Persistence: exerting effort despite setbacks
• Flexibility: changing attitudes and circumstances
• Optimism: viewing new opportunities as possible and attainable
• Risk Taking: taking action in the face of uncertain outcomes

One important goal orientation statement that can be conveyed to the student is that the future is full of unplanned events and so it is vital to see new ventures as adventures. The career coach can help to facilitate the student's learning "to create and benefit from future planned and unplanned events one step at a time" (Krumboltz, 2008, p. 147). The student's concern must be heard and seen to be heard, and it is equally important to get the student to share stories of past successes with unplanned events such that they can be enlightened to see that the lessons learnt be applied for the present or future. Even if the student is unable to recall past successes, past experiences can be reframed for reflection on what they could have done differently.

In Box 11.2, we look at a case illustrating the application of Krumboltz's (2008) HLT, where the career coach works with a student in SIT preparing for a work attachment, also known as Integrated Work Study Programme (IWSP).

Box 11.2   Case Study of Career Coaching for a Work Attachment Position

Leela was a second year Engineering student who was facing challenges in securing a position for the Integrated Work-Study Programme (IWSP). Tina, the career coach, observed that Leela felt socially awkward around people and would get anxious in crowded settings. Even in school, Leela interacted minimally with her peers. Her condition seemed to have restricted her options and she hoped Tina could advise how she could secure an IWSP position.

Tina used helping skills to connect with Leela and asked probing questions to clarify the challenges she had listed in her IWSP application. Leela was unable to secure a position after the first round of application when more than 60 per cent of her peers had succeeded. As Leela had limited time left, Tina prioritised working with Leela to research on other companies and roles, besides preparing her for interviews. After going through résumé consultation and mock interviews with Leela, Tina felt there was little progress as Leela did not do well in interviews and was still unable to secure an IWSP position. Tina took on the role of a buddy with some effort, after having established trust over ten or more sessions. She was able to clarify more of Leela's influences and learnings in her life journey. During the sessions, Tina gave Leela space to formulate her responses and to grow comfortable with long pauses. The subsequent sessions were heavily informed by Krumboltz's Happenstance Learning Theory: Tina helped Leela identify the possible environmental influences and associative learning from her journey. Leela shared her pre-university learning journey, which led to the formation and crystallisation of her interest in the renewables and sustainability industry.

Leela's family and friends felt that her career choice to be an engineer did not align with their belief that girls should be in female-oriented roles. However, Leela had positive role models in her secondary school teachers who took the road less travelled where they shared what they encountered and how they overcame the challenges when they did not accept the societal norms. Tina was reminded of a similar situation in her recent career transition and shared her story of embarking on an engineering career, so Leela knew that she was not alone and there are others who were in a similar situation. It was a vicarious moment for both Tina and Leela, which was a breakthrough that further strengthened their connection.

During subsequent sessions, Tina assured Leela that rejections are part of the job search journey, and to not overgeneralise the rejections to personal aspects of herself. She reminded Leela of her positive role models who stayed curious to explore learning opportunities and continued to upskill and learn throughout their careers. Tina noticed that Leela was beginning to feel more relaxed and spoke with greater affirmation. Leela initiated more sessions to do interview practice to prepare for her upcoming applications. She became more confident in pursuing her passion and considered a career in renewable energy.

In the case study, we saw how the student's social and familial influence had shaped her perception of her potential across the years, which was ameliorated by associative learning (which is learning through observations) across the months. The career coach played the role of a motivator and a counsellor using Krumboltz's (2008) framework and was able to inject optimism and flexibility into the student's mind, making her curious of her personal potential. This certainly took time, and the coaching process was an iterative one, but the student had that persistence in her to begin with, which was why she had sought the help of the career coach. By initiating more interview practices, the student showed that she was preparing to take risk beyond her comfort zone in the uncertainty of future interview chances.

The five Happenstance skills (optimism, curiosity, flexibility, persistence and risk taking) are important, and they allow one to cross the fine line that differentiates threats from opportunities. The student was empowered to pursue her passion and "take the road never travelled" (Krumboltz, 2008, p. 142). In the process, she showed that she could achieve more in life because of what she could do. It can be inferred thus that the actions she had taken would lead to "more satisfying career and personal lives" (Krumboltz, 2008, p. 135, 141), so the actions she took ought to be recognised and learnt well as they were born out of the Happenstance skills. It is important to remember that the goal is "not to make a single career decision" but for personal enrichment, so it is possible that the conscious choice made today can develop into another opportunity in future. Box 11.3 suggests some career coaching questions that can be considered.

Box 11.3   Some Career Coaching Questions from Krumboltz (2008)

1 Tell me what's on your mind.
2 How did you come to discover the activities that energise you?
3 Was there an event that influenced your life or career decision? ... How did that happen? ... What did you do after that?
4 What do you believe is stopping you from doing what you really want to do?
5 What do you think is your first step you could take now to move closer to what you want?
6 What is stopping you from taking that first step?
7 How would your life become more satisfying if you would take appropriate action?

Conclusion

This chapter identifies how career development theories are integrated into career education and coaching conversations. This integration is not merely theoretical but is applied practically, as can be seen in the employment of Schlossberg's Transition Theory (in identifying the transition factor to work on with the student) and Holland's RIASEC profiling tool (to clarify the student's doubt about their vocational choice). The examination of career development theories in practice highlights the dynamic nature of career coaching for different students' needs.

Furthermore, the discussion underscores the critical importance of a theory-informed approach in career coaching within higher education: this approach not only equips students with the necessary skills and insights for the development of their career paths but also prepares them to navigate the evolving landscape of work and life catalysed by technology. Krumboltz's Happenstance skills then become vital in a world of new practices transformed by artificial intelligence (AI). The student who stays curious, persistent, optimistic, flexible and takes risk is well positioned to take charge of their career journey in such a world. As career coaches, our role extends beyond immediate career guidance; it involves instilling in our students the resilience and adaptability required for lifelong personal and professional development.

Discussion Starters

• In addition to career coaches, who else in higher education can support students in making career choices?
• What are some methods or approaches you could use that will enable you to connect with your student effectively?
• How can you manage and motivate a student who does not follow through with his/her action plan?

- What would you do to coach a student who does not seem to take career preparation seriously?
- How can you support a student, weighed down by negativity and a fixed mindset, to use the Happenstance skills to move forward with their career-related decisions?

References

Braun, D. J. (2022). The experience of deep connection in coaching relationships. *International Journal of Evidence Based Coaching and Mentoring, S16*, 173–184. https://doi.org/10.24384/3tc6-ba81

Center for Credentialing & Education. (2023). *Core competencies: Global career development facilitator*. www.cce-global.org/credentialing/gcdf/corecomp

Conoley, C. W. & Conoley, J. C. (2009). *Positive psychology and family therapy: Creative techniques and practical tools for guiding change and enhancing growth*. John Wiley & Sons.

Cox, E. (2013). *Coaching understood: A pragmatic inquiry into the coaching process*. SAGE Publications. https://doi.org/10.4135/9781446270134

Evans, N. J., Forney, D. S., & Guido-DiBrito, F. (1998). *Student development in college: Theory, research, and practice*. Jossey-Bass.

Forward Singapore Workgroup. (2023). Chapter 2: Embracing learning beyond grades. *Forward Singapore*. www.forwardsingapore.gov.sg/-/media/forwardsg/pagecontent/fsg-reports/full-reports/mci-fsg-final-report_fa_rgb_web_20-oct-2023.pdf

Goodman, J., Schlossberg, N. K., & Anderson, M. L. (2006). *Counseling adults in transition: Linking practice with theory* (3rd ed.). Springer Publishing Company.

Government of Singapore. (2023). *Assessments*. My Skills Future. www.myskillsfuture.gov.sg/content/portal/en/assessment/landing.html

Hannum, K. M., & Hoole, E. (2009). *Tracking your development*. Center for Creative Leadership.

Holland, J. L. (1997). *Making vocational choices: A theory of vocational personalities and work environments* (3rd ed.). Psychological Assessment Resources.

Jordan, A. L., & Marinaccio, J. N. (2020). Career development theory and its application. In A. L. Jordan & J. N. Marinaccio (Eds), *Facilitating career development: An instructional program for career services providers and other career development providers* (Revised 4th ed., pp. 3–23). National Career Development Association.

Kohli, A. (2016). *Effective coaching, and the fallacy of sustainable change*. Springer International Publishing. https://doi.org/10.1007/978-3-319-39735-1

Krumboltz, J. D. (2008). The happenstance learning theory. *Journal of Career Assessment, 17*(2), 135–154. https://doi.org/10.1177/1069072708328861

Kunos, I. (2017). Role of coaching models. *International Journal of Research in Business Studies and Management, 4*(9), 41–46.

Mitchell, K. E., Levin, A. S., & Krumboltz, J. D. (1999). Planned happenstance: Constructing unexpected career opportunities. *Journal of Counseling & Development, 77*(2), 115–124. https://doi.org/10.1002/j.1556-6676.1999.tb02431.x

Ng, J., Yeo, M. -F., & Foo, Y. L. (2020). The integrated work study programme at Singapore Institute of Technology: More than a traditional internship model. In S. M. Lim, Y. L. Foo, H. T. Loh, & X. Deng (Eds), *Applied learning in higher education: Perspective, pedagogy, and practice* (pp. 17–26). Informing Science Press.

Schlossberg, N. K. (1984). *Counselling adults in transition: Linking practice with theory*. Springer Publishing Company.

Part IV

Leveraging the Potential of Coaching for Educators and Students

12 Coaching in a Student Support Programme

Bavani Divo, Fun Man Fung, Ramesh Shahdadpuri, Peng Cheng Wang and Eric Chern-Pin Chua

---

Chapter Objectives

- To share how some learning institutions initiate support programmes to develop students' metacognition and self-regulated learning skills to enable them to achieve academic and wellbeing goals.
- To explain why integrating coaching into a support programme initiative can create positive student impact.
- To discuss cases illustrating how coaching fosters students' self-awareness and metacognitive abilities within a support programme framework.

Keywords

coaching
growth mindset
learning approaches
learning journey
metacognition
motivation
self-regulated learning
self-regulation
wellbeing

Introduction

Beyond the formal curriculum, a repertoire of programmes seeks to develop students holistically in areas outside of academic content, such as metacognition, self-regulation and wellbeing. This chapter will draw attention to a cross-university collaboration for undergraduate students to use metacognition to plan, implement, assess and review their learning approaches as self-regulated learners. It also discusses how the integration of coaching in such a support

DOI: 10.4324/9781003332176-16

programme can significantly impact their self-regulation skills. This structured programme introduces students to setting SMART goals, crafting learning plans, the impact of sleep and learning, motivation and other self-regulation principles. After the small group facilitated sessions, coaches conduct individual coaching to generate solution-focused conversations and explore and apply manageable options to improve coping and wellbeing. Coaching enabled heightened awareness and use of metacognition for students to apply what was learnt in the programme and experience positive outcomes in their goals and overall wellbeing.

Importance of Supporting Students to Adapt and Thrive in University

Balancing life as a university student can be demanding, with increased expectations and more workload compared to when they were in high school or other pre-university programmes. Students may find it challenging to manage their time effectively, handle various types of assignments and adapt to the rigorous lifestyle as an undergraduate. Therefore, besides developing students' specialised knowledge and skill sets, a university education must also provide learning opportunities for their holistic development.

This includes nurturing soft skills, socio-emotional wellbeing skills and growth mindset, all valuable for self-management and workplace success. Employers expect students to be competent in communications, personal effectiveness and digital literacy, cutting across disciplines. Developing students' self-awareness, self-confidence, agility and resilience contributes to their positive wellbeing during university life as students and post-graduation.

How can soft skills be taught, growth mindset be cultivated and positive behaviours be encouraged within a university curriculum? Should they be part of the formal curriculum as credit-bearing courses? What about optional programmes beyond the standard curriculum, including offering extracurricular activities such as clubs, performing arts, sports and special interest groups?

This chapter shares two Singapore universities' efforts in developing and delivering programmes that aim to help students thrive by building on students' holistic development using metacognition as a foundation. The programme has also been adapted and implemented in a university in France (Institut Villebon Georges Charpak, n.d.). While each programme involves teaching students content that aims to develop them to become better learners, coaching was introduced in the process of helping students apply the content and explore actionable ways to be successful in their studies. The first part of the chapter provides an overview of these learning programmes, while the second section focuses on the coaching that took place.

Background of the Learning to Learn Better (LTLB) Programme

National University of Singapore (NUS): Where Learning to Learn Better Started and Grew

In 2017, the Institute for Applied Learning Sciences and Educational Technology (ALSET) at the National University of Singapore (NUS) launched its pilot of the elective module, Learning to Learn Better (LTLB), which was built to provide learners with the knowledge and practical strategies to help them succeed in the module of studies (Krishnan, 2018).

According to the past enrolment data, most NUS undergraduates graduated from junior colleges (JC) and polytechnics, encompassing certificates of pre-university equivalent to high school qualification in the Singapore education system. The transition from a curriculum-based to a modular system in NUS was challenging for many students. As a myriad of modules hosted at NUS provided differentiated paths for undergraduate education, it was important to teach learners how to learn to have the right skills to chart their learning journey (ALSET, 2018a).

In particular, the LTLB module was conceived to help students avoid common misconceptions about learning and develop evidence-based study practices. The module activities were designed based on examining the literature from the field of learning sciences (Fung & Kamei, 2019). In the face-to-face classes, the instructors demonstrated to learners using in-class experiments how best learning practices can sometimes be counterintuitive.

Since 2018, LTLB has been offered as a for-credit module structured via a blended learning experience by a series of 12 short instructional videos on key concepts in learning science, with reflective tasks and in-person seminars in which students work through the module learning outcomes. Students were invited to participate in related research studies (Yeo et al., 2021). The research findings suggested that late-type students (students who tend to be delayed in their behaviour or habits about academic activities and routines) have lower grades, less sleep and higher absenteeism.

The LTLB learning outcomes of the NUS programme are shown in Table 12.1.

Table 12.1 National University of Singapore: Learning to Learn Better Programme

Learning outcomes (LO)	Syllabus/topics
LO1. Assess their strengths and weaknesses critically in their prior approach to learning	• Collaboration • Goal setting
LO2. Identify, defend, and communicate learning strategies they use in other modules before and after	• Interleaving
LO3. Create their repertoire of self-selected learning strategies to enhance their learning independently	• Making connections • Managing sleep
LO4. Identify the characteristics of high-quality learning via the Science of Learning	• Practice • Repetition
LO5. Develop a personal plan and a learning philosophy based on self-awareness and understanding	• Self-motivation • Self-organising

The course was highly popular and enrolled nearly 900 students in one semester in 2020. The student feedback shed light on how well the module encouraged reflection on prior study techniques and the successful adoption of new learning strategies for enhanced academic performance. The feedback highlights a willingness to push oneself outside of one's comfort zone and break away from established study patterns, which eventually helps to improve learning outcomes and retention rates.

LTLB was subsequently adapted as a module for 83 working adults in the education sector in 2018 under the NUS Lifelong Learning Initiative for Alumni (ALSET, 2018b; Fung, 2019). During this run, LTLB mostly supported the educators in their professional development by presenting techniques for learning derived from a scientific understanding of how people acquire, process, and apply information and skills. In the module, the instructors taught the participants to reflect and incorporate effective and evidenced-based learning strategies into their educational programmes and classrooms to help their students learn better. Because of its reach locally and internationally, educators affiliated with NUS and SIT initiated deliberations concerning potential collaborative endeavours for the LTLB initiative. This initiative aimed to extend its educational influence across a broader spectrum of learners within the Singaporean context.

Singapore Institute of Technology (SIT): Collaboration of the Learning to Learn Better Programme

Singapore Institute of Technology (SIT) collaborated with NUS to adopt and adapt the LTLB programme. To support its graduates in their pursuit to thrive in their learning journey, the merits of the LTLB programme provide possibilities for valuable integration in SIT.

The LTLB curriculum at SIT is similar to that at NUS, but it strongly emphasises the "new normal" of learning that COVID-19 has introduced, which makes online learning elements much more prevalent than before. This adaptation entails a greater integration of aspects of online learning, including improved virtual learning skills and collaborative online participation. Table 12.2 documents the topics of SIT'S version of the programme

The Learning to Learn Better programme initiated in NUS was adapted, contextualised and tailored for the students of SIT to align the pedagogical approach of applied learning and learning objectives with the institution's distinctive learning environment and student demographics. Students in the programme are guided in using metacognitive processes to explore and learn learning strategies, unlearn ineffective learning methods and relearn approaches that can fulfil their goals. Increased self-regulated learning is related to goal setting, self-monitoring, self-evaluating, time management and motivation, which can bring academic success in higher education (Theobald, 2021; Wolters & Brady, 2020). This makes up the core content of the LTLB programme. The integration of individual student coaching was a key differentiator in the SIT LTLB programme.

Table 12.2 Singapore Institute of Technology: Learning to Learn Better Programme

Module topics	Subtopics
1. The Metacognitive Cycle	• Understanding metacognition • Applying metacognitive strategies
2. Setting SMART Goals for the Semester[a]	• Defining SMART goals • Boundary goals vs aspirational goals
3. Managing Time Effectively for Learning	• Time management techniques • Prioritising tasks and activities
4. Crafting Learning Plan for Study[a]	• Designing a personalised study plan • Incorporating study strategies
5. Memory and Retention	• Memory and its limitedness • Strategies for improving information retention
6. Staying Motivated for Learning	• Acknowledging successes and sources of motivation
7. Overcoming Challenges in Learning	• Identifying and addressing learning challenges
8. Learning with Others Effectively Online	• Developing a group contract • Establishing trust and effective partnerships

[a] See Appendix A.

Delivery of LTLB Programme in SIT

Students generally looking to improve themselves enrol in the Learning to Learn Better programme for 12 weeks in a semester. The programme also supports students facing academic probation, warnings or hurdles that inhibit them from bringing out their potential to be effective learners.

In the programme, instructors guided students through engaging discussions about various learning approaches and self-regulatory strategies, including finding a balance between enhancing learning and managing wellbeing. Each session was designed to focus on gearing students towards development through meaningful activities that enable them to reflect on their goals and learning plan, put their learning strategies to test and explore ways to motivate them in their learning.

Insights from student feedback and interviews highlighted a gap between students' knowledge attained through the LTLB sessions and implementing strategies learnt through one's daily learning and activities. While the LTLB programme provided a structured framework to facilitate students to learn about strategies to improve themselves, there was a need for an individualised avenue for students to be guided and explore solutions based on their unique situations and challenges. In pursuit of enhancing the implementation and effectiveness of student learning within SIT's LTLB programme, the introduction of coaching was implemented to create a greater impact and foster a more comprehensive learning support experience.

Coaching in the LTLB Programme

There is a lack of educational programmes that nurture students' metacognition and self-regulation. Many students are unprepared for effective learning using metacognitive processes and self-regulation (Howlett et al., 2021). Links between student success, metacognition and self-regulated learning (SRL) are becoming significant themes of academic research, programme innovation and higher education policy (Schunk & Greene, 2017). In addition to contributing to student success, coaching can be integral as it can reinforce institutional efforts to support students in their academic progress. Coaching in academic settings has gained increasing attention due to its association with improved study skills and academic performance, and has become a part of essential student support in universities (Capstick et al., 2019).

Students in the LTLB programme were each assigned a coach to work with to support their implementation of strategies to strengthen their self-regulation and metacognition. Coaches are introduced to students from the start of the programme, sharing their background and credentials to assure students that they are in good hands and that the coaches are there to support their journey to be effective learners. The coaches in the LTLB programme are SIT staff members who have attended the in-house coach training programme, "Coaching as An SIT Educator" (see Chapter 13).

The Roles and Expectations of Coaches and Students in the LTLB Programme

It is important to explain to the students that the coach's role is not like that of their academic instructors and programme lecturers. Coaches in the LTLB programme specifically journey with the students to enable them to translate their learning and takeaways into actionable plans. SMART goals and learning plans crafted by the students are used as a basis for coaching discussions, and notes (see Appendix B) are maintained in a confidential folder to carry on effective conversations with students throughout the programme.

The 1:1 coaching sessions were scaffolded to aid learners in identifying concrete solutions to better their learning journey and to help integrate knowledge and skills obtained from the LTLB programme in actionable ways in their daily lives. Coaching also makes it possible to closely explore workable strategies to empower learning, monitor progress, and provide encouragement and timely nudges.

The students in the LTLB programme come with little to no prior experience of being coached. Students learn content revolving around the concepts of self-regulation and wellbeing. During coaching sessions, students are expected to integrate the acquired content on self-regulation, wellbeing, time management and learning motivation within the taught metacognitive framework, applying these concepts actively in their daily learning routines. They are also expected to develop actionable plans applying knowledge gained through LTLB sessions.

Each student is strongly encouraged to complete the 1:1 virtual coaching sessions during the semester with their assigned coach over Zoom. The sessions are spaced out at least 3–4 weeks apart to allow students to implement their plans, experience their planned learning activities, and assess and revise their plans accordingly as they go along. Students are more likely to come on board and commit to coaching sessions when the discussions in these sessions are both meaningful and directly applicable to their experiences in the LTLB sessions, fostering a sense of relevance and practical implementation.

Coaching and Student Impact in the LTLB Programme

The programme has grown in the direction of adding value to students' learning of the original LTLB programme through a more holistic approach with coaching added. Without coaching, acquiring learning concepts and knowledge within the LTLB programme proves inadequate for fostering continuous growth and improvement. Conversely, including coaching in the LTLB programme leads to improved learning outcomes. As shown in Figure 12.1, students who attend LTLB sessions are provided with knowledge and skills to explore. They are then encouraged to complete developmental tasks such as goal setting, crafting a learning plan and writing reflections.

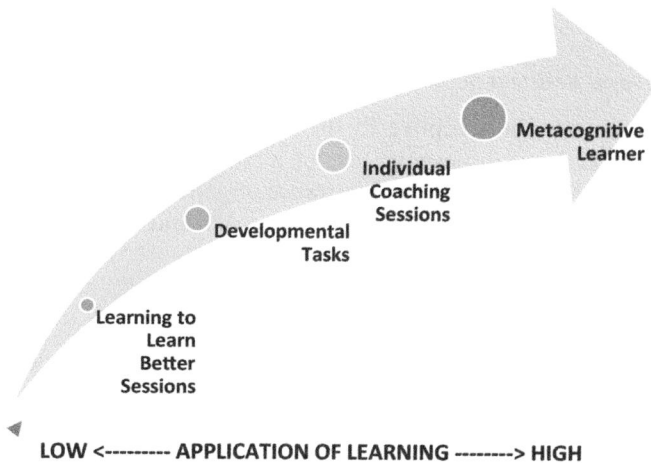

Figure 12.1 The student's journey in the LTLB programme

Coaching empowers students to develop practical ways to handle their learning obstacles and take significant strides to advance as learners in the LTLB curriculum. At the beginning of the programme, students are purposefully guided to identify personal goals and craft learning plans. They also write reflections that help shed light on challenges and concerns they may be facing.

Coaching facilitates deeper learning from LTLB sessions and higher tasks completed to experience progress as a metacognitive learner. When concrete, actionable plans are implemented during coaching sessions, progress is made as a learner. Learners are urged to apply their learning takeaways gained from LTLB at every step of the programme and learning journey. This includes application of learning during sessions, completing developmental tasks, participating in coaching sessions, and progressing towards becoming independent metacognitive practitioners. See Appendix A for developmental tasks assigned to students.

Coaching has served as a key feature in the success of the LTLB programme to reinforce the importance of self-regulation and metacognition as students strive to be better learners. Coaching helps foster accountability through check-ins beginning and mid-LTLB programme that help students manage their goals and plans. By supporting students in their self-regulation and metacognition through a personalised approach, coaching students is a crucial differentiator and positive value-add from SIT's earlier version of the LTLB programme.

Application of Coaching within the Programme

Drawing upon our accumulated experience, we present three illustrative vignettes to exhibit how coaching students can effectively generate positive impacts.

Case 1 – A Student Resistant to Coaching

Not all students may be receptive to the idea of being coached. In the first vignette in Box 12.1, we discuss the case of a student who initially resisted the idea of coaching. We highlight the importance of getting students on board and having a clear understanding of the roles of the coach and the student as coachee.

Box 12.1   A Student Resistant to Coaching

Vignette 1

VJ is a first-year Engineering student on academic probation. He wanted to attend the LTLB structured programme but was resistant to the idea of coaching as it was something he had not experienced before. The term was novel, and he doubts it might get him anywhere. His coach provided him with some context and explained how coaching could affect his learning journey. After two sessions of individual coaching, VJ stated that the coaching had motivated him to take concrete actions to make useful changes in his learning. He managed his time and workload better and did well enough to come out of academic probation. Coaching helped him in acting on his plans and become a more confident learner.

Suggested Coaching Questions

1 What motivated you to join the LTLB programme?
2 How do you feel about having a coach as your partner who supports you to achieve academic success?
3 From your list of SMART goals, which would you like to start working on first?
4 What changes could you make to be more focused on accomplishing your academic goals?
5 How will you monitor your progress towards your goals?

Reflection Questions for Coaches

1 How do I build rapport with the student and get him to understand how coaching can benefit him?
2 What steps can I take to support and motivate the student to be actively engaged in the coaching process?
3 How can my coaching build on the LTLB lessons to reassure and encourage the student to move forward?

In the vignette, the student needed to be made aware of what coaching was about as he doubted its impact on him as a learner. As coaches support students in their goals set and learning plan, after the first session, students can understand the coach's role better and recognise the tailored, personalised objectives of the sessions. This assures and instils confidence in the students to carry on with the coaching sessions, some even beyond the prescribed number of sessions in the programme.

The coaching conversations play an integral part in seamlessly linking coaches with learners. Goal-setting exercises and crafting of learning plans in the LTLB sessions serve as useful tools and focus points for conversations in the coaching sessions. Coaches enable students to develop a deeper understanding of their strengths and areas of improvement through these tasks and guide them through reflective solution-focused conversations to commit their plans to behaviour. When learners experience "what's in it for them" in the coaching sessions, they are more committed and meaningfully engaged in conversations with the coach.

The clear understanding of the roles of the coach and students from the programme's start affirm learners and promote students' willingness to adhere to coaching sessions. As learners are guided to focus on their challenges, plans and goals in the sessions, they gain confidence in coaching and their coaches. Coaches facilitate students to take steps to further the knowledge gained in the LTLB lessons and journey with them to realise concrete actions to take in their pursuit of being better learners.

Case 2 – A Student Struggling with Learning and Coping

It is frequently observed that students face challenges with their wellbeing when they are experiencing difficulties in managing their learning. Coaches in the LTLB programme are mindful of providing space and empathy for learners to explore ways of enhancing their learning experience without focusing solely on the mistakes students may have encountered during their educational journey. They put themselves in the student's shoes and understand students' challenging learning situations to provide guidance and steer coaching conversations aligned to support the students. Vignette 2 in Box 12.2 depicts a student struggling with learning and coping.

Box 12.2   A Student Struggling with Learning and Coping

Vignette 2

Nicky is a third year accountancy student struggling to balance his studies with his wellbeing. He was constantly experiencing burnout, having a negative outlook on life and questioning his purpose as a student. His academic performance declined over the semesters. He managed to cut down on the modules taken in the recent semester but still had consistent trouble managing stress and workload. He enrolled himself in the LTLB programme and was paired with a coach to journey with. By the end of the semester, Nicky achieved a balanced approach to time management, effectively scheduling breaks and maintaining a consistent rest and sleep routine. He shared with his coach the self-regulation habits he had created daily to enhance personal wellbeing helped him manage his learning better and he was less stressed.

Suggested Coaching Questions

1 How important is it for you to prioritise your wellbeing?
2 With respect to your wellbeing, on a scale of 1 to 10 (with 1 being very low and 10 being excellent), where are you now? Where would you like to be ideally (a follow-up question after the coachee responds to the first question)?
3 Which aspects of your wellbeing would you like to discuss in this coaching session?
4 What steps can you take to get enough daily rest and sleep to improve your wellbeing?
5 How will you know if your plan to overcome burnout and improve wellbeing is working?

Reflection Questions for Coaches

1 What can I do to help the student understand that self-regulation affects personal wellbeing and enables him to be an effective learner?
2 How do I demonstrate empathy in my coaching conversations to support students struggling with their workload and stress?
3 How can I have open, non-judgemental conversations with students who are hesitant to share their wellbeing challenges and ways to improve?

In the vignette, Nicky's experience was due to poor time management over the semesters. As a result, Nicky constantly struggled with deadlines and was studying until the last minute, which brought about a state of burnout. Nicky's time was always used up to catch up on learning and he had minimal opportunities to take a proper break and prioritise his wellbeing. He was not getting enough sleep, staying up late to complete projects and assignments. Nicky's coach helped facilitate conversations that enabled Nicky to develop actionable plans for improvement. The coach demonstrated high levels of empathy by encouraging Nicky to find solutions while staying on track with the established goals. This provided a safe space for Nicky to explore options to manage his time better and improve his stress management. Nicky experienced positive morale and motivation as the coach reinforced his small steps toward success.

Students typically expressed experiences of being challenged by the rigour of their studies and difficulties keeping up with their learning plan. Consequently, coaching conversations focus on enhancing the learning plan and implementing necessary adjustments. Within the framework of metacognition for reflection, coaches scaffolded conversations concerning both successful and less successful aspects of the past weeks. Students then explored ways to tweak the learning plan to implement the following week and were closely monitored to identify areas of difficulty for further review. This process helps students develop metacognitive skills and become more aware of their learning processes. Topics on motivation, time management, sleep, memory retention and working effectively with peers learnt in the LTLB programme are discussed to refine their skills, address challenges, and achieve higher levels of success.

Habit-building timelines are discussed to help minimise disruptive habits. Coaches in the LTLB programme take the opportunity to understand individual students better through these conversations. Acknowledgement and encouragement are given to reinforce students' concrete actions to achieve their short-term goals. Providing words of affirmation on their progress, regardless of the results, is also crucial in bolstering student motivation. For instance, a slight adjustment in sleep patterns to attain more restful hours is acknowledged and supported within the coaching session to reinforce the positive action taken by students to better his wellbeing. While the goal may relate to improving wellbeing, coaching is action-oriented and empowers students to study and improve wellbeing proactively.

Empathy serves as a driving force for change in others. Empathy supports learners to think deeply about their motivations and feelings and share them with the coach (Watson et al., 2013). Coaching conversations are kept open and friendly to put students at ease and coaches practice active listening to understand their perspectives fully. Coaches have shared that responding to student sharing and discussion points with empathetic language helps build trust and rapport. Demonstrating empathy through acknowledging and validating students' experiences avoids having a judgemental and critical lens of students' shortcomings, paving the way for insightful and constructive solution-focused coaching conversations. It is pertinent for coaches to demonstrate empathy while maintaining objectivity and staying focused on the students' intentions during the conversation. This also strengthens the coach and learner in building a more productive relationship (Wolff et al., 2019).

Case 3 – Developing Growth Mindsets

Coaching offers excellent opportunities for students to develop growth mindsets as they discuss challenges and solutions to overcome them. Through

---

Box 12.3   Developing Growth Mindsets

Vignette 3

Sky is a final-year hospitality student doing her best to keep up with her studies. However, she constantly feared experiencing failure and often was uncertain about her abilities to keep developing herself as a learner. During a project assignment, she encountered difficulties keeping up with her teammates and was constantly caught up in negative self-talk. She enrolled in the LTLB programme to gain tips on developing a growth mindset. Peer sharing in LTLB sessions and coaching conversations encouraged her to take small steps to cultivate positive-self talk. The "Change Talk" activity enabled her to process her thoughts and reframe her thinking (see Appendix C). She completed the programme successfully and stated that it would help pursue her career proactively and that she experienced a boost in motivation at various junctures to keep her moving forward purposefully. Her sustained motivation enabled her to stretch beyond her comfort zone. With the coach's support, she was able to overcome minor setbacks in her life, remind herself of the effort and progress she had made, and continue to work on them. She aims to thrive in her academic pursuits while enhancing her growth mindset through active participation in self-development activities.

Suggested Coaching Questions

1 When faced with unfamiliar tasks, how do you usually approach them?
2 How can you use reframing (such as "Change Talk") to shift your perspective and foster a growth mindset?
3 How would you seize growth opportunities so that you can continuously learn and develop your capabilities?
4 What strengths do you possess that would enable you to persevere in the face of challenges on your pathway?
5 Which aspects of yourself would you like to work on to perform better and achieve excellence?

Reflection Questions for Coaches

1 How do I have coaching conversations to encourage students to embrace challenges and view failures as opportunities for growth?
2 What can I do to help students develop belief in themselves to explore opportunities beyond their comfort zone in their learning journey?
3 How can I inspire students to recognise their strengths to support them, to perform from good to better, and better to excellent?

coaching conversations, coaches can help students see the value of a growth mindset in university and their daily lives post-graduation. A growth mindset is an asset for any learner, by enabling students who are struggling to take gradual steps to improve, to move on from any failure and for students who are striving to advance towards excellence.

In the vignette presented in Box 12.3, Sky benefitted from the LTLB programme and coaching by believing in continuous learning and growth even when she is doing well in her academics. She can apply her learning and growth mindset in the working world to continue to improve herself. The coach was able to stretch Sky's potential and discussed opportunities for her to explore ideas outside of her comfort zone. Coaching sessions helped reinforce tips and knowledge gained in the LTLB programme and reframe setbacks. By scaffolding and guiding to break difficult tasks down to manageable bite-sized steps and completing them progressively, it boosted motivation and empowered Sky to embrace challenges and celebrate her wins.

Coaches in the LTLB programme leverage on resources used in the classroom sessions to encourage learners to adopt the growth mindset. Students in universities can benefit from a growth mindset intervention, with particular attention to goal setting, reflecting on failures and effort-based coping. Adopting a growth mindset has direct implications on student success (Sorensen, 2016). Learners in the LTLB programme have varying degrees of fixed and growth mindset that surface during coaching conversations. Coaches can encourage students to explore ways to embrace and reinforce a growth mindset, preparing them for lifelong learning beyond their time at university. To experience progress in their learning journey, learners must believe in their capacity to improve. Inculcating a growth mindset can empower students to embrace failures and continue to learn and improve their ways in all aspects of their life.

Based on the self-determination theory, autonomy, competence and relatedness are key driving forces to intrinsic motivation (Deci & Ryan, 2012). Coaches can help to identify learners' strengths, leveraging them to foster competency and facilitate success. In coaching sessions, learners can lead and choose what topics they want to discuss and work on. As a result, students take ownership of the actionable plans that they formulate and can be motivated to carry out what they had planned. As coaching sessions revolve around students' needs and plans, students can relate and connect with the content at a deeper level. In addition, when coaches support students to help them realise their potential, it can serve as a boost in motivation to help students move forward.

Coaching in the LTLB programme also provides opportunity for students to discuss and understand their motivation and demotivation factors, reminding them of what they can do to keep moving forward. A coaching conversation sheet as shown in Appendix B can be helpful for note taking. The coaching conversations build on student tasks completed in the class sessions, such as the "Change Talk" sheet (Appendix C), which help to identify areas they need to reframe, reconstruct and rewire to experience progress.

Conclusion

Integrating coaching within a student support programme, brings about positive student outcomes. Through the structured programme, students can learn from their instructor and peers on content related to effective learning and wellbeing. The coaching allows individualisation and holds students accountable to take action on what they have learnt. Learning from a support programme is more enriched when paired with coaching focused on students' metacognition and self-regulation. As students learn to trust their journey with coaching, and work towards achieving their goals in concrete ways, their metacognition and self-regulation develop, which paves the way for future successes. With coaching, students are in charge of their learning, monitoring and cyclically adjusting their plan according to the learning outcomes and developing self-efficacy through this discovery process.

Discussion Starters

- Imagine your role as a coach within a university support programme. How would you prepare yourself to actively engage and effectively support students?
- How do you envision the shift from being an educator to becoming a coach, and what kind of mindset do you believe is necessary to embrace this transition?
- Coaches often encounter unique challenges when working with students. What are the potential challenges you might face when implementing a

student support programme (such as Learning to Learn Better) at your university?
- Who would be the key stakeholders and supporters you need to work with in your organisation to develop and implement a student support programme (such as Learning to Learn Better)?

Acknowledgement

We acknowledge the funding support from the MOE TRF Grant, "MOE2020-TRF-013" (MOE TRF Supporting Academically Weaker Students by Improving their Self-regulation for Online Learning) for this collaboration between SIT and NUS under a specific Research Collaboration Agreement.

We extend our sincere appreciation to the Institutional Review Board (IRB) of the Singapore Institute of Technology (SIT) for their support throughout the research process. Their thorough review and registration of this study ensured its ethical compliance and adherence to the highest standards of research integrity.

Appendix A Developmental Tasks

Task	Objective	Coaching Session
SMART goals	To identify goals for the semester that are: • Specific • Measurable • Achievable • Relevant • Time-bound	The coach utilises SMART goals as a tool to initiate conversations that facilitate planning and progress towards the objectives.
Learning plan	To guide students to achieve goals set	The coach utilises the student's learning plan to address successes and areas for improvement, fostering a discussion on enhancing future actions.
Letter to self (reflection)	To empower students to recognise their challenges and accomplishments, fostering self-awareness and motivation for continued personal growth and perseverance.	The self-reflection is exclusively reviewed by the instructor and subsequently returned to the student upon the programme's conclusion, serving as a recollection of their past, present, and journey.
Change talk (reflection)	To pinpoint obstacles hindering students' progress and engage in reflective practices to formulate strategies for addressing these challenges in the future.	The coach utilises the "Change Talk" reflection to comprehend the areas in which the student seeks improvement, thus facilitating conversations aimed at modifying thought processes.

Appendix B Coaching Conversation Sheet (For Coach's Notes)

Coach:
Coachee:
Date:
Time:

1. Coaching goal for the session:

2. Action plan in brief:

3. Strategies and practices in learning:

4. Notes on student's progress towards SMART goals and learning plan:

5. Notes on student's self-regulation (efficacy, motivation):

6. Notes on student's wellbeing:

7. Any other notes/comments:

Appendix C Sample of "Change Talk" Reflection

Change Talk	Reflection	Self-Reflection Question
"I'm really struggling with this my project work. I keep thinking that I'm not good at it.I have to make efforts to develop my abilities."	I realised I needed to positive self-talk to remind myself of the importance of putting it effort and hard work to be better.	What small steps can I take each day to positive self-talk??
"I can't keep fixating on my failures every time I cannot do as well as I wanted."	I realised I compare myself to peers and get discouraged.	How can I focus on my efforts and personal growth?
"I can't keep avoiding tasks that are out of my comfort zone."	I realised that I need more guidance in writing academic reports for my projects.	Whom can I reach out to for a discussion about this, and who can guide me towards finding the necessary support?

References

ALSET (2018a, June 14). *Learning to learn better for NUS alumni – What do they learn in our course?* [Video]. YouTube. www.youtube.com/watch?v=JQ19pl6ZrMA

ALSET (2018b, June 21). *ALS1010 learning to learn better (what is it?)* [Video]. YouTube. www.youtube.com/watch?v=PpwtLG_L6uA

Capstick, M. K., Harrell-Williams, L. M., Cockrum, C. D., & West, S. L. (2019). Exploring the effectiveness of academic coaching for academically at-risk college students. *Innovative Higher Education, 44*(3), 219–231. https://doi.org/10.1007/s10755-019-9459-1

Deci, E. L., & Ryan, R. M. (2012). Self-determination theory. In P. A. M. van Lange, A. W. Kruglanski, & E. T. Higgins (Eds), *Handbook of theories of social psychology: Volume 1* (pp. 416–437). SAGE Publications. https://doi.org/10.4135/9781446249215.n21

Fung, F. M. (2019). *Learning to learn better!* Projects Platform. Retrieved 19 December 2023, from https://projects.directory/projects/LFv5b24F/summary

Fung, F. M., & Kamei, R. K. (2019). How blended learning in tandem with team-teaching help learners improve performance in *"Apprendre a Apprendre!"*

Howlett, M. A., McWilliams, M. A., Rademacher, K., O'Neill, J. C., Maitland, T. L., Abels, K., Demetriou, C., & Panter, A. T. (2021). Investigating the effects of academic coaching on college students' metacognition. *Innovative Higher Education, 46*(2), 189–204. https://doi.org/10.1007/s10755-020-09533-7

Institut Villebon Georges Charpak (n.d.). *Partenariats de recherche.* www.villebon-charpak.fr/experimentation-pedagogique-2/partenariats-de-recherche/

Krishnan, K. R. R. (2018). *The art of learning: Learn to learn.* Institute for Application of Learning Science and Educational Technology (ALSET).

Schunk, D. H., & Greene, J. A. (2017). Historical, contemporary, and future perspectives on self-regulated learning and performance. In D.H. Schunk & J.A. Greene (Eds), *Handbook of self-regulation of learning and performance* (pp. 1–15). Routledge. https://doi.org/10.4324/9781315697048-1

Sorensen, C. E. (2016). *The relationship of growth mindset and goal-setting in a first-year college course* [Master's thesis, South Dakota State University]. Open PRAIRIE. https://openprairie.sdstate.edu/etd/687/

Theobald, M. (2021). Self-regulated learning training programs enhance university students' academic performance, self-regulated learning strategies, and motivation: A meta-analysis. *Contemporary Educational Psychology, 66*, 101976. https://doi.org/10.1016/j.cedpsych.2021.101976

Watson, J. C., Steckley, P. L., & McMullen, E. J. (2013). The role of empathy in promoting change. *Psychotherapy Research, 24*(3), 286–298. https://doi.org/10.1080/10503307.2013.802823

Wolff, M., Morgan, H., Jackson, J., Skye, E., Hammoud, M., & Ross, P. T. (2019). Academic coaching: Insights from the medical student's perspective. *Medical Teacher, 42*(2), 172–177. https://doi.org/10.1080/0142159x.2019.1670341

Wolters, C. A., & Brady, A. C. (2020). College students' time management: A self-regulated learning perspective. *Educational Psychology Review, 33*(4), 1319–1351. https://doi.org/10.1007/s10648-020-09519-z

Yeo, S. C., Lai, C. K. Y., Tan, J., & Gooley, J. J. (2021). A targeted e-learning approach for keeping universities open during the COVID-19 pandemic while reducing student physical interactions. *PLOS One, 16*(4), e0249839. https://doi.org/10.1371/journal.pone.0249839

13 The Coaching Journey

Pathways for Institutions and Educators to Build Coaching Competencies and Culture

Ramesh Shahdadpuri, Cheryl Pei Ling Lian and May Sok Mui Lim

Chapter Objectives

- To understand what resources and actionable plans an educational institution needs to develop versatile coach–educators and create a sustainable coaching ecosystem.
- To appreciate the journey of a coach developing from novice to competent, and excelling to attain a recognised professional coaching credential.
- To evaluate how coaching benefits educators by achieving personal satisfaction and professional meaning through creating learning impact and transforming the lives of their students.

Keywords

change agent
coach–educator
coaching circle
coaching competencies
coaching culture
coaching ecosystem
coaching supervision
community of practice
mentor coaching
reflective practice

DOI: 10.4324/9781003332176-17

Introduction

Technology-driven disruptions and socio-economic shifts are having a significant impact on higher education. Digital tools and virtual platforms have become the norm for teaching and learning. From a traditional student base of young undergraduates, universities now have many adult learners who want to acquire new skills and qualifications to help them remain relevant in their jobs, pursue opportunities in promising growth sectors and achieve self-actualisation goals.

Educators in higher education must adapt to the new realities, which requires a mindset shift to deal with greater diversity and complexity. They cannot merely be classroom instructors in the traditional mold. They have to become versatile educators, adept in working with students to help them excel academically and to bring out the best in them to realise their full potential. Besides having teaching skills, educators must also be equipped with coaching capabilities to engage students in coaching conversations. As versatile coach–educators, they can be change agents who inspire students to make the best of opportunities for a rewarding university experience.

The Role of Coaches in Academic Settings

There are various perspectives on what is coaching in education. Academic coach is a commonly used term with different connotations (Robinson, 2019). One view is what an academic advisor does in helping students navigate their study path, such as choosing a major, completing prerequisite and elective courses, and meeting credit requirements for graduation. Another interpretation is that of a subject specialist tutor, such as in mathematics, who provides remedial help to students who need extra support for a course. Another perspective of academic coaching is performing the hybrid functions of academic advising and life coaching, helping students with study skills, time management, action planning and general wellbeing. In whichever way the term is used, there is general agreement that academic coaches in a university environment support students to organise themselves better and be more effective in managing their time and energy so that they excel in their academic performance and maintain good emotional wellbeing (Deiorio et al., 2017).

In this chapter, the authors use "academic coach" to mean "coach–educator". A "coach–educator" is any faculty and teaching staff who takes a coaching approach, using coachable moments in the classroom and other settings to have coaching conversations with students in individual or group situations. Coach–educators can work with students in broad areas, such as developing their interpersonal skills, professionalism, self-advocacy, and organisational skills (Wolff et al., 2019). Coaching students for learning is most effective when it incorporates evaluating performance, providing feedback, identifying gaps, creating goals, exploring solutions and holding students accountable (Deiorio et al., 2017). Coaching is a working partnership where learners have to take responsibility for their effort, be open with their coach–educator and participate meaningfully to make progress and improve performance (Lovell, 2017).

In educational institutions, coaching can overlap with the functions of teaching, advising and mentoring, all of which support students in some positive way. A key distinction is that when coaching students, a coach–educator is intentional about using a coaching approach and relies primarily on non-directive communications, mostly "asking" rather than "telling" or "giving advice". In coaching conversations, the coach–educator asks thoughtful and timely questions to get students to think and reflect, enabling them to come up with ideas, solutions and choices without being prescribed answers (Lovell, 2017). For academics to become coach–educators, they must be equipped with basic coaching capabilities. Training educators to develop foundational coaching competencies is essential to ensure baseline quality and consistency in their coaching approach (Deiorio & Juve, 2016).

Coach Training for Educators

The following section is helpful for readers considering implementing coaching in their institutions. To persuade key stakeholders and decision-makers, it is important to be clear about the "why" and "how" – the purpose and proposed steps for implementing the coaching initiatives. As faculty members are the leading players who interact with students, providing them with basic coach training is essential to become coach–educators.

There are different ways for an institution to get started with training. One is to offer optional coaching workshops which interested educators can sign up for. However, for coaching to become widely adopted in the institution and create a positive impact, coach training should be made mandatory for all educators, either as part of a teaching induction programme or professional development training,

Many training vendors can provide good coach training. However, their content tends to be skewed toward executive and leadership coaching for corporate clients. For training that delivers practical value for educators, it is essential to customise the contents to suit the higher education context. Hence, finding a suitable partner to design and contextualise coach training for academic settings is critical. An alternative training option is to build internal coaching capabilities within the institution. One way is to send university staff for professional coach training to earn an industry-recognised credential. Another choice is to hire a credentialed and experienced coach to manage in-house coach training and other coaching initiatives.

In Box 13.1, we share the story of our university's coaching journey as a case study. We hope that readers can learn about the prospects and challenges of such an undertaking and inspire those planning to take their first step in building a coaching ecosystem for their institutions.

Box 13.1   Case Study – Building Internal Capabilities for Coach Training in a University

Background

Singapore Institute of Technology (SIT) started its coaching journey with the belief that coaching students is aligned with its pedagogy and its aspiration to become a premier university of applied learning. The university leadership was willing to commit resources for faculty training to develop the coaching capabilities of its educators. Educators play a critical role in their interactions with students, being enablers and change agents in supporting students to have a holistic university experience and achieve academic success, personal growth, and general wellbeing.

The Coaching Journey Begins

SIT's Centre for Learning Environment and Assessment Development (CoLEAD) is responsible for implementation of best practices in teaching, learning, assessments, instructional design, educational technologies and providing general support for academic staff. CoLEAD was tasked to lead the university's coaching effort. In its initial attempt, CoLEAD worked with external training vendors. The course structure and materials were contextualised with relevant educational content. However, after working with two different vendors, the training outcomes did not meet expectations. CoLEAD then decided to pivot and develop its own coach training capabilities.

   A decision was made to hire an experienced coaching training specialist who would develop and deliver a new educator-focused coaching workshop and drive other coaching initiatives in SIT. The new coaching workshop, "Coaching As An SIT Educator", would be mandatory training for all teaching staff.

Planning and Delivering an Impactful Educator-Focused Training Programme

Coach training is most effective when it combines theory and practice using mixed methods, with elements of didactic instruction (lecture-based), skills training (demonstration and practice) and experiential learning (exercises, simulations and scenario role-playing) (Martin et al., 2013). Creating effective coach training can draw on the experience of other helping professions like social work and therapy, incorporating principles of instructing, modelling, rehearsal and feedback (Teding van Berkhout & Malouff, 2016). The course must cover the key coaching competencies and incorporate reflective practice to develop self-awareness, discernment and flexibility, preparing the leaners to engage in reflexive conversations and become effective coaches (Leggett & James, 2016).

An important element of the SIT training was incorporating the solution-focused approach. Solution-focused coaching is characterised by its simplicity and time effectiveness, shifting the coachee's focus from the past to using the conversational time for discovery of positive resources, hopes of a preferred future and constructive action steps to move forward (Grant & Gerrard, 2019). When educators engage in solution-focused dialogue, they can coach students to develop self-awareness of their thoughts, emotions and actions, and to work on their strengths and opportunities towards positive future outcomes.

The design of the two-day workshop, "Coaching As An SIT Educator" (Lim et al., 2023), incorporated ideas and concepts from relevant academic literature and professional coaching best practice, including coaching competencies and code of ethics. Key elements of content and learning activities included:

- Core coaching competencies (knowledge, skills and abilities) based on the International Coaching Federation professional framework (International Coaching Federation, 2019)
- Coachable moments in SIT (educators identifying learning opportunities with students)
- Solution-focused approach and emotional intelligence (awareness, empathy and positivity)
- Non-directive approach of coaching (versus other helping roles of teaching, advising, mentoring and counselling)
- Students' learning and development needs in SIT (academic performance, personal growth, workplace learning and career readiness)
- Relevant examples in academic settings (case studies and scenarios customised for SIT)
- Practice-focused with coaching roleplay sessions (with trainer and peer feedback)
- Formative assessment using scenario-based coaching roleplays with standardised students (with feedback by experienced observers)
- Reflective practice (self-reflection exercises and group sharing)
- Digital content for pre-workshop preparatory work (flipped classroom)

For further details on the coaching workshop, please see the Appendix.

Besides relevant content, designing a practice-focused workshop was an important consideration. Allocating time for coaching practice, with the trainers and peer learners in a psychologically safe space, would give participants opportunities to demonstrate their coaching competence. Feedback and feedforward from peers and observers, and interludes for reflective practice, would help consolidate learning. Identifying blind spots and areas of improvement, with recognition of what went well and receiving encouragement, would enable participants to build confidence and demonstrate progress in their coaching.

Assessment drives learning and it was important to include individual formative assessment. Towards the end of the second day, each participant has to do two short scenario-based coaching sessions with standardised students. Observers would be present to assess the participant's ability to conduct a coaching conversation and demonstrate key skills such as active listening, showing empathy and asking open questions. They are given individual feedback by the observers, which they can learn from and take forward as they continue to practise their coaching skills. The workshop concludes with reflection and discussion on what coach–educators can do to further develop their coaching skills.

Creating a Sustainable Coaching Ecosystem and Organisational Coaching Culture

There are other learning activities besides attending courses and workshops. For an organisation to embrace coaching, promoting regular coaching conversations and coaching practice is needed beyond introductory training workshops. Connecting with peers within the organisation and through wider professional networks can offer rich learning opportunities. Digital resources and sharing platforms with vibrant communities can make learning fun and engaging. When these resources are purposefully curated and organised around the theme of coaching in an organisation, they can be a catalyst for promoting coaching practice, nurturing a coaching culture and supporting continuous learning and professional development.

In Box 13.2, we continue from the earlier discussion and share SIT's continuous learning initiatives beyond the coaching workshop.

Box 13.2   Building a Coaching Ecosystem

Shortly after the launch of the two-day coaching workshop, a coaching community of practice was initiated. A community of practice involves a group of people sharing a common interest in a topic, getting together to learn more, with opportunities to explore deeper and learn from the other participants. The real value of such learning communities comes from a sense of belonging, creating new knowledge, sharing best practices through regular participation, and achieving individual and group learning goals (Wenger, 1998).

This coaching community of practice, called "Coaching Conversations @SIT", reinforces the lessons learnt in the coaching workshop and functions as a peer learning platform. It promotes discussions and collaboration around coaching knowledge and practice, exploring coaching topics and research from practitioners and academics (Deiorio & Juve, 2016). The monthly SIT community meetings are hour-long virtual sessions open to all SIT educators. Participating members are invited to propose topics of interest and volunteer to facilitate sessions on coaching topics of their interest. They are raising awareness and promoting collective learning to help sustain curiosity and support for coaching practice and developing a coaching culture in the university.

With the success of the community of practice, an extension of this learning format was launched. "Coaching circle" is an active learning forum where real coaching cases are discussed. Coaching circles involve deeper engagement and understanding of challenging coaching issues, making it a more intense learning experience (Brassard, 2019). Each session is led by case protagonists who share their experiences handling real-life and challenging coaching cases. The personal details of the coachees are not disclosed. Through questions and dialogue with participants, the case unfolds. The protagonists can challenge the circle participants to give their perspectives and suggestions on what they would do if they were in the coach's shoes. The discussion concludes when the case protagonist reveals what happened in the case without violating anyone's privacy, and the facilitator summarises key takeaways from the case discussion.

Besides the workshop, a community of practice and a coaching circle, the other pillar in SIT's coaching ecosystem is a knowledge repository. Named "Coach Academy", it consists of digital resources that anyone in the university community can access if they want to learn more about coaching. It is updated regularly, with reference lists and resource links for access to relevant academic sources, professional coaching literature and other industry resources. The repository contents are organised into four categories for easy user search: General Coaching Resources, Coaching Knowledge & Practice, Coaching Science, and Coaching in Education.

Mentor Coaching and Coaching Supervision for Continuous Learning

A motivated coach who wants to take his coaching practice to a higher level can look for opportunities to work with and learn from experienced coaches. Mentor coaching and coaching supervision are learning relationships highly encouraged by the professional coaching associations for their members undergoing coach training and clocking their learning hours for continuous professional development.

Mentor coaching involves working with a more experienced mentor coach so that the mentee coaches can sharpen their knowledge, build confidence in applying the coaching competencies and learn about current topics relevant to their coaching practice. For example, the International Coaching Federation describes mentor coaching as a mentor coach partnering with mentees to develop a deeper understanding and practical insights related to the ICF Core Competencies, including the Code of Ethics (Passmore & Sinclair, 2020). The mentor coach also reviews mentees' coaching situations with clients, including coaching observations and recordings, sharing feedback and distilling lessons learnt to increase the mentee's coaching capability. Guiding mentees in reflective practice is an integral part of the mentoring process, helping them to develop greater self-awareness, recognise strengths and areas of improvement, and thoughtfully use the time and space during mentoring to explore ideas to become better coaches. Mentor coaching takes place over an extended period, allowing the mentees to show steady progress. Mentor coaching can be done in group and individual sessions.

Another impactful learning path is coaching supervision with an experienced coach supervisor. The Association for Coaching in the UK describes coaching supervision as "a formal and protected time for facilitating a coach's in-depth reflection on their practice with a trained Coaching Supervisor" (Hawkins et al., 2019, p. 5). Unlike our common understanding of the word, supervision in coaching is not about hierarchy or policing. It is a professional relationship based on trust and collegiality. There are similarities to mentor coaching, including dialogue-based collaborative learning and reflective practice. However, the main difference is that mentoring emphasises mastering the coaching competencies, while supervision focuses on other aspects of the supervisee's coaching. This includes the supervisor reviewing the supervisee's internal coaching process, ethical issues, blind spots, biases, areas of improvement, and any other tangible and psychological issues, helping the supervisee gain clarity and insights about their inner self (International Coaching Federation, n.d.)

Hawkins et al. (2019) see the coach supervisor's role, when working with the supervisee, covering three areas:

1 Qualitative function – increasing the quality of the work being done by the supervisees with their clients and client organisations.
2 Developmental function – helping the supervisee's continuing personal and professional development, grow their capacity and continually learn from the challenges encountered in their practice.
3 Resourcing function – increasing the supervisee's capability to work from their source rather than physical effort, sustaining self and the coaching practice, and increasing their capacity for creativity and resilience.

The three functions are interlinked and reinforcing. As a coach develops, they grow in their capacity to resource themselves, thereby increasing the quality of their work (Hawkins et al., 2019).

An Overview of the Professional Coaching Arena

For coach–educators, their coaching capabilities can make them more effective in their work as academics and positively impact their students. Some of our university coach–educators have expressed interest in coach training at a higher level. For any interested novice, the next step would be to attend a training programme for professional coaches. This section overviews the professional coaching industry and helps readers understand more about pursuing further training and professional credentialling.

From a global perspective, the most well-known professional coaching bodies are the Association for Coaching (AC), the European Mentoring and Coaching Council (EMCC), and the International Coaching Federation (ICF). These coaching associations all aim to promote the professionalism of their members and establish high standards by building trust through professional best practices and ethical codes of conduct. Each has credentialling requirements and processes to ensure members receive and attain the minimal training needed to be competent coach practitioners. These associations also offer valuable networking and training resources to advance coaching knowledge, skills and best practice. They lead discussions on the latest developments and emerging trends to benefit members and the wider community. Table 13.1 gives an overview of the major coaching professional bodies.

Table 13.1 Overview of the Major Coaching Professional Bodies

Professional Body	*Association For Coaching (AOC)*	*European Mentoring & Coaching Council (EMCC)*	*International Coaching Federation (ICF)*
Year founded & head-quarters	2002 United Kingdom	1992: United Kingdom 2002 (Reconstituted): Belgium	1995 United States of America
Membership (end–2022)	Above 7,000	Above 10,000	Above 50,000
Countries/ territories represented	Over 80	Over 85	Over 140

(Continued)

Table 13.1 (Continued)

Professional Body	Association For Coaching (AOC)	European Mentoring & Coaching Council (EMCC)	International Coaching Federation (ICF)
General Information	A leading independent, not-for-profit professional body dedicated to promoting best practices and raising the awareness and standards of coaching worldwide. Its purpose is to inspire and champion coaching excellence, to advance the coaching profession, and make a sustainable difference to individuals, organisations and society.	A voluntary, not-for-profit providing coaching and mentoring professional accreditation, support and guidance to the coaching and mentoring profession, and its members. It represents the profession within the European Union and globally. It has created a range of industry standard competency frameworks, rules and processes for coaching, mentoring and related supervision. It works with many private and public sector European organisations on coaching and mentoring qualifications, accreditations, code of ethics and frameworks.	A non-profit organisation for fellow coaches to support each other and grow the profession. In 2020, it changed its name from the International Coach Federation to the International Coaching Federation, to reflect a new way of serving coaches, coaching clients, communities and the world, with a vision of coaching as an integral part of a thriving society. In 2021, it unveiled a new ICF brand and "One" ICF ecosystem, represented by six unique family organisations, reflecting ICF's interests in many areas of the coaching industry.
Website	www.associationforcoaching.com	www.emccglobal.org	www.coachingfederation.org

From Novice to Competent: Pursuing Further Training for Coaching Advancement

A novice coach–educator who wants to attain higher coaching proficiency will have to go for advanced training at the professional level. It is commendable to pursue a professional credential, and it will be a challenging journey, exploring deeper into the coaching competencies and engaging in hours of deliberate practice, which requires a commitment of time and financial resources (Hullinger & DiGirolamo, 2020).

Each professional coaching body's credentialling criteria is different with respect to the stipulated training requirements, minimum practical coaching hours, and professional ethics assessment. Selecting which professional credential and training pathway to pursue is an individual choice. Factors to consider include where one is based, which coaching body is most recognised in that jurisdiction, and personal preference.

This chapter has mostly discussed the coaching journey from an institutional perspective. This section tells a personal story of an SIT educator's coaching journey. In this vignette, Cheryl talks about her path from taking the two-day basic workshop run by the university to pursuing a professional coaching credential. She signed up for a professional coaching training programme, which will lead to an ICF credential upon completion. Cheryl's story is in Box 13.3.

Box 13.3   A Coach's Journey

Introduction

I am Dr Cheryl Lian, Assistant Professor in the Health and Social Science cluster at the Singapore Institute of Technology. In February 2021, I enrolled in the "Coaching as An SIT Educator" workshop led by ICF-certified SIT faculty coach Ramesh, as part of my continuous professional development. I hoped to arm myself with fundamental coaching knowledge and strategies, which seemed to be a natural extension of improving direct communication with my students.

The workshop turned out to be both inspiring and transformative in my mindset, where the immediate benefit was an increased awareness of my teaching presence in the classroom, with a strong emphasis on a learner-centred dialogue approach. Essentially, this approach involves a coach conversing with his coachee using the GROW framework and getting the coachee to:

1 Identify and set a **G**oal (this may take up the most time in a single session since goals may or may not immediately be apparent to the coachee),
2 Do a **R**eality check,
3 Consider various **O**ptions available, and finally,
4 Find a **W**ay forward.

I learnt that the four basic steps could be applied iteratively and implemented in a cyclical fashion throughout the coaching conversation to lead the coachee to uncover personal insights. In essence, this simple framework of dialogue was a useful methodological approach to raise my students' awareness levels and to arm them with the confidence to move ahead, even in the face of roadblocks, by generating possibilities.

I feel that with the two-day intensive workshop, I was very much equipped to apply my newly acquired coaching knowledge and skills to empower my learners to identify what it was that really mattered to them to move forward. As a novice coach practitioner, this was the beginning of what a "solution-focused" coaching approach meant to me – a very simple, powerful, practical and coachee-focused way of empathetic communication to help my coachee reach the desired outcome by way of increased awareness and by relooking at existing circumstances from a different perspective, through the gentle art of dialogue. One of my favourite tools is the scaling technique to help my coachee gain greater perspective and self-management by avoiding oppressive problem-centred talk and focusing on the possible way forward by drawing on previous successes and existing resources to reach the end goal.

A Coaching Example

My student (coachee) was feeling overwhelmed, from juggling multiple personal commitments to coping with the ongoing demands of school-work. He made an appointment with me to discuss his progress. My intention for the session was to help my coachee to see beyond his challenging circumstances and to consider what was already going well for him. With this reframed state of mind, I hoped that my coachee could get in touch with what was truly important to him and leverage his identified strengths and previous successes as his source of intrinsic motivation to overcome current difficulties.

This is a sample coaching conversation snippet where I intentionally applied the scaling technique to raise my coachee's self-awareness and promote deeper reflection.

Me (as coach): On a scale of 1 to 10, with a score of 10 referring to being wildly successful at finding a balance in managing your multiple commitments and 1 being the opposite of that, where are you now?

Coachee: (After a long pause) I would rate myself at a 4 in finding balance – overwhelmed, distracted and unsuccessful on most days.

Me: What have you done to reach a level 4 and not any lower?

Coachee: Looking back on how I have come this far, I would say that I have been lucky to have had the renewed opportunity to pursue my degree despite coming from a troubled family background from my younger days. While I am feeling overwhelmed now, I have to say I have mostly been able to bounce back from difficult situations.

Me: Thank you for your sharing. Where on this scale would you like to be, and what would it look like for you?

Coachee: I would say 7. At level 7 of my reimagined life, I would feel a lot calmer – I would not be as distracted as I am now, my anxiety is currently getting in the way of my ability to focus on the task at-hand, that is, to participate actively in class and get more out of my education.

At this point, I did not hesitate to commend my coachee for his resilience and forwardness in the conversation. For the remainder of our session, I continued to use coaching techniques to draw upon and centre his awareness on existing and past successes. Ultimately, my coachee recognised that to overcome this difficult period in his life required small, actionable steps that he desired to implement daily. My coachee acknowledged that if such consistent changes were to be made, we needed a way to track individual progress. We decided to have a follow-up session where outcomes could be reported. This though would not be a mandatory session. The coachee would be at full liberty in deciding if he wanted coaching to continue or if the conversation had already paved his way forward.

Taking Coaching to a Higher Level

As I look back, I am fascinated by how solution-focused coaching, an unhurried, no-nonsense method, applied to the student being coached, kept me grounded in the belief that all learners have the potential for positive change. I knew that at my very core as an educator, I wanted to take my personal development a step further by enrolling in an ICF-accredited training programme that would provide me a structured pathway to becoming a certified coach. Building on the foundational principles that the solution-focused coaching workshop at SIT had afforded me, I was confident I would most certainly be able to deepen and extend the application of this method to all aspects of my professional and personal life.

I am currently midway through my journey towards becoming a solution-focused coaching "expert". I have gained much in terms of being introduced to the various dialogic models and toolkits available (such as SCAMPER, SCORE, BRIEF and OSKAR models) to become a more effective and enlightened coach practitioner, by empathetic listening, and selecting and building upon my coachee's dialogic sharing. I have had many practice sessions in my external coaching masterclass where all attendees further help me strengthen my coaching skillset with constant dialogue sessions. I particularly enjoy the reflection that comes along with carefully analysing dialogic conversations. In my journey towards becoming a coaching expert, I have gained heightened personal awareness as to what extent the conversation between myself (as a coach) and coachee is solution-focused. Using the three constituents of empathy intervention, goal intervention and strategy intervention during a typical 30-minute coaching conversation leads to constructive solution-focused talk in a non-directive, pragmatic and holistic way.

I must admit that coaching is grounded in mindfulness and awareness, a trait too often overlooked amidst our hectic lives. A particularly fascinating aspect which I want to deepen my coaching skillset in is on the aspect of appreciative inquiry which can be further applied to team coaching. To quote my professional coach mentor Simon Lee, "behind every problem, there is a wish". By making use of what is already there (the client's previous experiences and resources), we can make a difference to our client's outcomes by widening their perspectives through raising awareness and generating possibilities.

My opinion is that it is indeed time for all formal beginner teacher professional courses and higher education staff training to incorporate coaching mindset as a foundational basis for continuous professional development, just as how SIT has successfully done. It is imperative that educators equipped with the coaching skillset can more effectively help our individual learners maximise their potential.

Coach the Person, Not the Problem

Coaching is often described as a partnership where the relationship is coachee-centred. The coach offers support by giving time and space for the coachee to take responsibility for generating ideas, establishing goals and committing to action. Novice coaches tend to focus more on the coaching process, especially when asking questions and using coaching tools learnt in training. The novice coach may approach the coachee's immediate issues at the surface level and have them set goals and action plans expeditiously. While this can support the coachee to arrive at solutions, coaching that creates real impact must go deeper.

A more experienced coach would have a stronger coaching mindset and greater coaching presence, with the acuity and confidence to holistically appreciate the coachee's needs. A seasoned coach possessing greater awareness, curiosity and intuition can notice shifts in the coachee's speech, emotions and behaviours. As a thinking partner, the coach creates trust, openness, and a safe space, being non-judgemental and intentional about coaching the whole person, not just the problem (Reynolds, 2020). The coach guides the coachee to navigate from the inside out, provoking critical thinking and challenging assumptions and beliefs. The coachee can move towards positive change and transform their life with greater awareness and insight.

A coach who sees the coachee as a whole person and works with them at a deeper level for transformational coaching is a change agent. A coach who is fully present and intentional in the service of the coachee can be said to be "dancing in the moment", being open and adept to the new directions and developments of the coachee.

> Coaches are dancing in this moment when they are being completely present with the client, holding the client's agenda, accessing their intuition, letting the client lead them. When coaches dance in the moment, they are open to any steps the client takes and are willing to go in the client's direction and flow.
>
> (Kimsey-House et al., 2011, p. 175)

The Joys and Rewards of Coaching

Socrates said, "Virtue is its own reward". Coaching is a virtuous endeavour in which the coach uses his capabilities to support, influence and inspire others to become a better version of themselves. The act of coaching is a virtuous cycle as it brings benefits to the coaches too. When speaking to coaches, they share that they notice positive changes in themselves as others do when they have become coaches. This includes communicating better by listening more and talking less, having higher emotional intelligence, greater equanimity, stronger intuition, better powers of observation, greater self-confidence, more clarity of purpose, gratitude and humility. Coaches also say that coaching others has made them more patient and caring, curious and open-minded, non-judgemental and appreciating others' strengths. Their coaching journey has given them more exposure and widened their social and professional networks, contributing to their personal growth and development.

For coach–educators, using their coaching capabilities together with their expertise and talents as academics gives them great influence in shaping the lives of their students. Educators are drawn to the profession for many reasons, including the opportunity to develop people through teaching and the satisfaction of seeing students grow and transform. These strong intrinsic motivators give educators a deeper sense of purpose, self-worth, inner joy and career satisfaction. Educators can remember the individual students that they coach well because of the relationships built and the rewards of witnessing their students grow. Educational institutions must commit to and support the development of coach–educators and coaching ecosystems to navigate the path forward in a rapidly changing educational landscape. Harnessing the synergy of being a "coach" and "educator" can raise the quality of teaching and the student learning experience.

Conclusion

Higher education is undergoing massive disruption with rapid technological change and greater diversity and complexity as more adult learners and mid-career professionals seek to attain degrees and professional certifications. In this new reality, the way educators engage students must change. Educators must develop new capabilities in coaching and be trained in the basic coaching competencies to become "coach–educators". The training for educators must cover more than generic coaching content and be contextualised for academic settings, delivered by experienced coach trainers who understand the educational context.

As coach–educators, they can have coaching conversations with students whenever coachable moments arise, within and outside class hours, in formal or informal settings. A coaching approach can support students to excel in their academic performance, personal growth and general wellbeing. Staff who are novice coaches and are motivated to learn more can be encouraged to attend advance coaching training. They can follow the training pathway of professional coaches and earn a credential awarded by a recognised coaching body.

The university can consider investing resources to develop its in-house training capabilities for coaching impact and sustainability. Beyond training workshops, building a wider university coaching ecosystem, such as communities of practice and coaching circles, is important. Learning from peers and experienced coaches through mentor coaching and coaching supervision are highly effective ways to grow and develop as a coach. All these initiatives and platforms can collectively contribute to building a coaching culture to drive the institution forward.

Discussion Starters

- As an educator, how do you manage your multifaceted role with students and perform the tasks of instructor, advisor, mentor and coach?
- If you want to learn more about coaching, who would you approach in your professional and social circles to discuss this? What would be some questions you would ask that would help you to gain useful insights?
- Suppose you have no coaching experience and find out that your organisation supports sending you for coaching training. What is your current level of interest in pursuing this opportunity based on a scale of 1 to 10 (where 1 = very little interest and 10 = very high interest)? Why did you choose this number?
- What is your experience of participating in a live or virtual interactive communal learning platform such as a community of practice? If you were to organise and lead a community of practice in your organisation, what guidelines would you put in place to ensure it is successful?

Appendix Overview of SIT's In-House Coaching Training Workshop

Workshop: Coaching as an SIT Educator

Learning Outcomes

By the end of this course, participants will be able to:

1. Articulate the role and responsibilities of a coach/mentor in educational settings.
2. Demonstrate listening, questioning and feedback skills to have good coaching conversations.
3. Apply the GROW coaching model to conduct coaching sessions.
4. Show empathy to build rapport and foster good relationships.
5. Implement coaching/mentoring in academic and workplace attachment settings to achieve the desired programme outcomes.

Topics Covered

Pre-Workshop: eLearning

- Mindset & Motivation
- Emotional Intelligence (EQ)
- Feedback Skills
- What Is Coaching?

Workshop:

- Coaching & Mentoring Fundamentals
- Coaching Tools & Techniques
- Mentoring
- Getting Feedback On Your Coaching
- Summary & Closing

Assessments

Role Plays: Standardised Students & Assessors Scenarios (each – 20 minutes):

1. Academic context
2. Workplace attachment

Quiz: Multiple Choice Questions (MCQs)

- Emotional intelligence
- Building rapport & trust
- Coaching conversations
- Coaching process: GROW Model
- Role of educator-coach

References

Brassard, C. (2019, April 1). *Coaching circles: Leveraging coaching skills in a truly inspiring environment.* International Coaching Federation. https://coachingfederation.org/blog/coaching-circles

Deiorio, N., & Juve, A. M. (2016). Developing an academic coaching program. *MedEdPublish, 5,* 143. https://doi.org/10.15694/mep.2016.000143

Deiorio, N. M., Skye, E., & Sheu, L. (2017). Introduction and definition of academic coaching. In N. M. Deiorio & M. M. Hammoud (Eds), *Coaching in medical education: A faculty handbook* (pp. 1–5). American Medical Association.

Grant, A. M., & Gerrard, B. (2019). Comparing problem-focused, solution-focused and combined problem-focused/solution-focused coaching approach: Solution-focused coaching questions mitigate the negative impact of dysfunctional attitudes. *Coaching: An International Journal of Theory, Research and Practice, 13*(1), 61–77. https://doi.org/10.1080/17521882.2019.1599030

Hawkins, P., Turner, E., & Passmore, J. (2019). *The manifesto for supervision.* Association for Coaching and Henley Business School. https://cdn.ymaws.com/www.association forcoaching.com/resource/resmgr/home/manifesto_for_supervision_20.pdf

Hullinger, A. M., & DiGirolamo, J. A. (2020). A professional development study: The lifelong journeys of coaches. *International Coaching Psychology Review, 15*(1), 8–19. https://researchportal.coachingfederation.org/Document/Pdf/3496.pdf

International Coaching Federation (2019, October). *Updated ICF coaching competencies*. (Accessed: May 10, 2023). https://coachingfederation.org/app/uploads/2021/03/ICF-Core-Competencies-updated.pdf

International Coaching Federation (n.d.). *Coaching supervision*. (Accessed July 1, 2023). https://coachingfederation.org/credentials-and-standards/coaching-supervision

Kimsey-House, H., Kimsey-House, K., Sandahl, P., & Whitworth, L (2011). *Co-active coaching: Changing business, transforming lives* (3rd ed.). Nicholas Brealey Publishing.

Leggett, R., & James, J. (2016). Exploring the benefits of a coach development process... on the coach. *International Journal of HRD Practice, Policy and Research, 1*(2), 55–65. https://doi.org/10.22324/ijhrdppr.1.116

Lim, S. M., Shahdadpuri, R., & Pua, C. Y. (2023). Coaching as an educator: Critical elements in a faculty development program. *The Asia Pacific Scholar, 8*(2), 70–75. https://doi.org/10.29060/TAPS.2023-8-2/SC2802

Lovell, B. (2017). What do we know about coaching in medical education? A literature review. *Medical Education, 52*(4), 376–390. https://doi.org/10.1111/medu.13482

Martin, B. O., Kolomitro, K., & Lam, T. C. M. (2013). Training methods: A review and analysis. *Human Resource Development Review, 13*(1), 11–35. https://doi.org/10.1177/1534484313497947

Passmore, J., & Sinclair, T. (2020). *Becoming a coach: The essential ICF guide*. Springer Nature. https://doi.org/10.1007/978-3-030-53161-4

Reynolds, M. (2020). *Coach the person, not the problem: A guide to using reflective inquiry*. Berrett-Koehler Publishers.

Robinson, J. A. (2019). *Community college success coaching: A phenomenological exploration of an emerging profession* [Doctoral dissertation, Baylor University]. BEARdocs. https://baylor-ir.tdl.org/items/22bc603c-9f81-4ca8-a00f-c57fdba4d3e6

Teding van Berkhout, E., & Malouff, J. M. (2016). The efficacy of empathy training: A meta-analysis of randomized controlled trials. *Journal of Counselling Psychology, 63*(1), 32–41. https://doi.org/10.1037/cou0000093

Wenger, E. (1998). *Communities of practice: Learning, meaning, and identity*. Cambridge University Press. https://doi.org/10.1017/CBO9780511803932

Wolff, M., Morgan, H., Jackson, J., Skye, E., Hammoud, M., & Ross, P. T. (2019). Academic coaching: Insights from the medical student's perspective. *Medical Teacher, 42*(2), 172–177. https://doi.org/10.1080/0142159x.2019.1670341

Index

Pages in *italics* refer to figures and pages in **bold** refer to tables

Printed and bound by CPI Group (UK) Ltd, Croydon, CR0 4YY

27/11/2024

01796051-0004